PORTFOLIO CAREERS for GPs

The countless hours I spent writing
this book would not have been
possible without God and my family.
For that I will be eternally grateful.

PORTFOLIO CAREERS for GPs

HOW TO BUILD YOUR IDEAL CAREER AND IMPROVE YOUR WORK–LIFE BALANCE

Patrice Baptiste

MBBS, BSc (Hons), MRCGP
Portfolio GP, London, and Senior Lecturer at the University of East London

Scion

© **Scion Publishing Ltd, 2024**

ISBN 9781914961564

First published 2024

Scion Publishing Limited

The Old Hayloft, Vantage Business Park, Bloxham Road, Banbury OX16 9UX, UK

www.scionpublishing.com

Important Note from the Publisher

The information contained within this book was obtained by Scion Publishing Ltd from sources believed by us to be reliable. However, while every effort has been made to ensure its accuracy, no responsibility for loss or injury whatsoever occasioned to any person acting or refraining from action as a result of information contained herein can be accepted by the authors or publishers.

Readers are reminded that medicine is a constantly evolving science and while the authors and publishers have ensured that all dosages, applications and practices are based on current indications, there may be specific practices which differ between communities. You should always follow the guidelines laid down by the manufacturers of specific products and the relevant authorities in the country in which you are practising.

Although every effort has been made to ensure that all owners of copyright material have been acknowledged in this publication, we would be pleased to acknowledge in subsequent reprints or editions any omissions brought to our attention.

Registered names, trademarks, etc. used in this book, even when not marked as such, are not to be considered unprotected by law.

Typeset in India by DataWorks
Printed in the UK
Last digit is the print number: 10 9 8 7 6 5 4 3 2

Contents

Why I wrote this book: my story   vii
Acknowledgements   xiv

1: Introduction   1
  1.1 What is a portfolio career?   1
  1.2 Why might it be good to consider a portfolio career? 3
  1.3 What challenges might you face when creating a
     portfolio career?   4
  1.4 Why are portfolio careers important now?   4
  1.5 Traditional GP roles and the portfolio career   6
  1.6 How this book can help you   8

2: Planning for a portfolio career   11
  2.1 The importance of career development in medicine   11
  2.2 Are you ready for a portfolio career?   12
  2.3 The first steps to developing your career   12
  2.4 The importance of assessing your interests, skills,
     qualities and achievements   14
  2.5 Understanding how time and the wider environment
     impact your career   22

3: Setting yourself up for career success   29
  3.1 Defining what career success looks like to you   29
  3.2 How can you achieve career success?   31
  3.3 How to assess your qualifications and work experience 38
  3.4 Self-help tools for successful career planning and
     development   47
  3.5 Identifying what additional support and (social) skills
     you need to stand out   52
  3.6 How your organisation can help you   72

4: A practical template for creating your career   81
  4.1 Categorising your portfolio   81
  4.2 How to actually get started, including some financial
     and legal aspects to consider   90
  4.3 Time management and balancing workload
     (including how to stay sane!)   95
  4.4 Goal setting   97

Why I wrote this book: my story

Before we get into the detail of how you can develop *your* portfolio career, I felt that it would be helpful for me to explain what prompted me to develop *my* portfolio career. I think that understanding my story will help you understand where you are now and how you can get to where you want to be.

Disillusionment

There I was, at a crossroads. Not sure where to go; I was stuck. Unfulfilled. Disillusioned. How did this happen… to me?

Ever since I can remember I wanted to work as a doctor. For years I relentlessly pursued this dream. Then one day it happened.

Finally completing my training, after six long years at medical school, I was ready to do what I signed up for. I was ready to help people using the knowledge and skills I had worked tirelessly to acquire.

However, it was not this straightforward. I was in for a huge shock.

Despite shadowing the doctors on the wards for three years as a medical student I was in no way prepared to start working as a doctor. There was so much I did not know. I am not referring to medical knowledge, because I expected that it would be a steep learning curve, and I knew that I would not give up and so learn all I needed to know to competently work as a foundation doctor and then as a specialty doctor. What I am referring to is the poverty of technology, the lack of staff, the lack of support for staff, the bureaucracy. I could go on. I was not taught any of this at medical school. In many ways I felt heartbroken. It was like unrequited love!

At the time I sensed that I had to make a decision: do I stay in a system that felt almost impossible to work and thrive in as a doctor? Or do I cut my losses, focus on transferable skills, and run whilst I still can? I was in my mid-20s, early on in my career; so, was it better to leave now than carry on miserable and living a lie? A portfolio career could offer the ideal balance, but seemed difficult to start whilst in full-time training due to the demands of training, exams and assessments. Creating a portfolio career, in my opinion, is much easier to do if part-time or when training is completed.

As medical students many of us leave medical school without enough training in the non-clinical aspects of a medical career (our finances, employment contracts as examples). We are therefore not really ready to develop our careers to the fullest extent possible. This lack of training, along with limited support for our mental wellbeing, can begin to lead to disillusionment and burnout. Starting to look for help in career development is an important step in starting to think about a portfolio career, and creating a career that really suits us. A career that we enjoy reduces disillusionment and burnout, and might just help improve retention and lead to better patient care and health outcomes!

So where can you learn the skills you need to develop your career? The British Medical Association (BMA) is obviously a good starting point, particularly its career development courses in the *Learning and development* section of the website (www.bma.org.uk/learning-and-development). In addition, you could look at Medschool Xtra (www.medschoolxtra.co.uk), a platform I created to help users (particularly medical students and early career doctors) assess their level of career readiness and to also learn much of the crucial knowledge needed to feel ready to start their careers. Finally, your more experienced colleagues will be able to help answer specific questions and guide you in the right direction.

The realisation

After the foundation programme, like many doctors do now, I took a FY3 or Foundation Year three as it is known. I took time out to essentially find myself (again) and decide what I was going to do. I had stopped literally all the hobbies and interests that made me happy and allowed me to destress and unwind. I used to write poetry but stopped that as there was no time. I used to read but stopped that too as my eyes were often too heavy and dry when I returned home. I used to love exercising but I stopped that because as soon as I sat down for a few minutes and had something to eat, just the thought of exercising made me tired again. It was a vicious cycle and it had to end somewhere. I had to stop it.

> Have you cut back on your hobbies and interests and started to feel that this might be a problem? Have you considered how you might find time to take them up again? If so, then a portfolio career might be a part of the solution.

I took that year to do all the things I used to enjoy. I also started networking. I hope you take away more from reading this book, but if you take just one thing away then make it that: network. The saying is true (as you may know already in your quest to get into medical school), "your net worth is your network". I networked at medical and non-medical events. I spoke to lawyers, accountants, writers, basically anyone who was not a medic. I learnt about their careers and absorbed all I could. I did attend medical events too and, surprisingly, I found out I was not alone. I felt very alone, but through the events I realised this problem was bigger than me. There were many doctors who felt like me, who were unsure about what to do. I felt sorry for those doctors who had mortgages and families to support because they felt so trapped. They had to provide for and support their loved ones even if that meant being unhappy and sacrificing their dreams. Many doctors did not even know what their dreams were any more. Many were not sure about what they would do if they left medicine; they were institutionalised. They had no idea who they were any more. That saddened me and I really felt for them. I am thankful that I was able to take the time to listen to my inner voice and realise that I still wanted to be a doctor. I still wanted to help people and become the doctor I had envisioned as a child. If I was ever going to leave and change careers, this was not the right time for me to do so.

Once I realised that I still wanted to work as a doctor I had to decide:

- Whether or not I could face returning to the NHS and, if I did, how I would survive. I would certainly have to find a way to become even more resilient (the buzzword that seems to be used more and more in medicine recently).
- If I returned, what would I do?

I decided that I needed to prepare myself mentally and emotionally for returning to what I felt was a broken system. Some of the things that I found helpful were writing down my long-term goals to motivate me (e.g. 'becoming a GP', 'financial security', 'career autonomy'), especially when things did not seem to be going to plan; I used exercise as an outlet which really helped when I returned to GP training after a long stressful day at work; I practised mindfulness to keep me focused and calm.

I decided that working in general practice was, for me, the best solution to the dilemma I was facing. GPs seemed to have more control over their careers, they had more variety both in clinical and non-clinical worlds, and in many cases they were able to build long-lasting and meaningful connections with their patients. They also seemed to have time for teaching students. At the time, most of the GPs I met, although under pressure, seemed happy with their choice of career. Therefore, I felt that general practice would enable me to have more career autonomy and ultimately become the doctor I envisioned.

The start of my portfolio career

That is when it began. I made a promise to myself that I was not going to let the system take away my passions again. I spent my FY3 year writing lots of articles – I enjoyed writing and wanted to develop my skills. I also wanted to incorporate it into my portfolio career somehow. I started writing poetry again because I found it therapeutic. I started a medical careers company (what I hoped would become a social enterprise, called DreamSmartTutors) and helped to support the next generation of doctors, and in the process developed as an entrepreneur, learning lots about the world of business. I knew it was going to be hard but I kept that promise to myself, and my portfolio career was born.

Once I returned to training, I did my best to continue what I started during my FY3 year. My portfolio career naturally happened, instead of being rigidly planned. I was still finding my feet in terms of becoming a GP, writer, speaker and so on. I spent several years working in these areas of interest, honing my skills. I felt it would be some time before I could say I have made a career out of them, or now have a portfolio career.

This is how it all started…

Working as a clinician

Once I completed my training, I started working as a salaried GP. Towards the end of my GP training I secured a job at a practice local to me. I then went on to work remotely as a locum. I was planning to stay at that practice for a long time because I was not keen on moving around, like I did during my training years. I really liked working there but I found it difficult to return to work after maternity leave. The pandemic also seemed to impact the dynamics at the practice, and returning to work almost seemed like returning to a completely different practice. I thought about continuing to work as a remote GP because I was not sure about returning to face-to-face work – I was concerned about losing my clinical skills but wanted to prioritise my wellbeing and my family. I took on a salaried role as a remote GP but felt that the pay was not sufficient for the significant workload, and left this role after about five months.

I returned to working remotely as a locum and, when the surgery no longer needed my services (one of the drawbacks to locum work!), I decided that it might actually be time to return to face-to-face working and managed to secure a long-term locum post at another local surgery. I earned more working in the surgery and was able to keep up my clinical skills. I had also started to feel slightly isolated working remotely (despite the efforts from the various surgeries to include remote GPs) and my son was growing up, so I felt it was a better time to try to make that transition.

Working as an educator

During my time in my first salaried post, I spent two years teaching medical students as a GP Tutor, and I completed courses to become a foundation trainee, out-of-hours and clinical supervisor. This led me to successfully undertaking a module on the Health Professions Education MSc at University College London (which helped me to secure several positions such as a GP educational fellow and senior lecturer at the University of East London). I also started examining medical students at Queen Mary University of London during my final year as a GP trainee.

I worked as a senior clinical lecturer at The College of Medicine and Dentistry, Ulster University (I didn't apply for this role, but was contacted by the CEO of the college via LinkedIn – I cover the importance of social media in *Section 3.5.3*!) and was appointed as an Associate Lecturer at The Open University.

I became registered as a PLAB (Professional Linguistic Assessments Board) examiner during 2019, which I applied for because it seemed interesting, and I wanted to gain experience in this area.

Working as an entrepreneur

As mentioned above, I founded DreamSmartTutors to enable me to deliver courses and workshops for those interested in a medical career. My main focus was to inform students about working life as a doctor so that they truly understood the realities of a medical career. I also aimed to improve diversity (in the form

xii Why I wrote this book: my story

of ethnicity and socioeconomic background) at medical school. Sadly, DreamSmartTutors ended for a number of reasons including wanting to focus on my family more, lack of a team and support as an entrepreneur. Later (see below) I started another entrepreneurial venture which was unplanned!

And, as I write this section, this is where I am now…

I have had to write this section of the book last because my career has changed significantly since I accepted the challenge to write this book, just over two years ago now. At the time of writing this book I am working in the following roles:

- Clinician – I work as a locum GP in a lovely practice, currently two sessions a week, potentially increasing to four sessions or starting as a salaried GP if a position arises. I also work remotely 1–4 sessions a month.

- Medical educator – I work as a senior lecturer and module lead at the University of East London. I occasionally examine OSCEs at Queen Mary University of London. I also run a YouTube channel (www.youtube.com/c/drpbaptiste) which focuses primarily on supporting those interested in and working in general practice; my patient information videos on here led me to being recognised by YouTube as a credible source of health information.

- Researcher and entrepreneur – along with my team at Medschool Xtra I am working on a tool to assess career readiness among medical students and early career doctors and provide them with the resources to enable them to become career-ready. I was accepted onto cohort seven of the NHS Clinical Entrepreneur Programme and received funding from the Medical Protection Society (MPS) Foundation for this work.

- Writer – working on this book! This has meant I have written fewer articles than in the past, although I continue to write for GP Online.

- Speaker – I speak at schools and colleges about a medical career, and also at universities and conferences about a variety of topics including career readiness and how to create a portfolio career (!)

What I really like about portfolio careers is the autonomy; they can change as much or as little as you want – you control the direction of your career. My career moves have been a combination of wanting to put my family and wellbeing first, alongside choosing what I think would be best for my career goals overall. Having a portfolio career has enabled me to make these changes. I am not reliant on one income and can supplement my main sources of income with smaller freelance roles such as speaking and writing.

Having a portfolio career does require some level of fearlessness and you have to be confident in taking risks, whether big or small. At times I have made what could be considered by some as quite drastic or hasty decisions, but I did what I thought was best at the time and, importantly, had the flexibility in my career to be able to do so.

In creating my portfolio career, I did not have access to a specific guide or framework. Everything I did was literally trial and error! Looking back, it would have been useful to have some more support and structured guidance in what could work and how to go about carving a portfolio career. Therefore, this book has been designed to support you as you begin your own journey to creating a portfolio career. It can be used as a practical guide based on research around career development, my own personal experiences – what has worked and not worked for me – and the stories of other portfolio GPs doing some amazing things. I truly hope it helps you find fulfilment and peace in your very own portfolio career!

Acknowledgements

The publishers and I would like to thank all the interviewees and interviewers who contributed to *Chapter 6*. The interviewers are a combination of medical students and doctors who are interested in general practice and/or portfolio careers. They were matched to the interviewee based on their interests and passion to learn more about a particular portfolio career. They were keen to participate in contributing, which would also help with their own career development.

I would also like to thank Scion Publishing for the opportunity and the much-needed support they provided along the way.

Chapter 1:
Introduction

As I described in the preceding pages on "Why I wrote this book", my portfolio career arose out of a desire to keep my hobbies and interests alive. You might be able to relate to this, or you might simply want to explore other career options that complement your current medical career. In this chapter we will explore a background to portfolio careers and end with how you can use this book to help you create your very own portfolio career.

1.1 **What is a portfolio career?**

Anyone who has multiple careers, jobs and interests has a portfolio career. These careers can be in different fields or they can be related to one field. In other words, there can be one primary career which acts as a foundation for other careers. For example, the foundation to my portfolio career (my main career or job) is working as a GP. However, there are many possibilities; the sky really is the limit. Importantly, a portfolio career can also include unpaid or voluntary roles (for instance, I was a school governor for four years), and it might be these that help keep some of your external interests alive.

'Portfolio working' or 'the portfolio life' was first described in the 1990s by Charles Handy, an author and social philosopher. He recognised that the world of work was changing and that it would be possible for individuals to juggle multiple jobs and interests, taking control of their income and wellbeing. One could argue that portfolio careers within medicine have always existed; Ctesias was a Greek physician and historian, whilst Saint Luke was a physician who was believed to have written two books in the New Testament. Other prominent doctors were Avicenna (mathematician, scientist, philosopher and poet) and Girolamo Fracastoro, the physician and poet who wrote about syphilis.

Fast forward to the present day – examples of doctors with portfolio careers include Atul Gawande (surgeon, public health researcher and author), Rosena Allin-Khan (A&E doctor and MP), and Zoe Williams (GP and media doctor).

So, whilst portfolio careers have seemed to become more popular, or more common among GPs, doctors across various specialties have for centuries balanced multiple careers and interests along with their clinical work.

Take a minute to reflect on:

- What made you pick up this book?

- Is there something missing in your life and/or current career?

- What would you like to spend more (or less) time on?

- Your career(s) and interests

- From reading about the doctors above, would you like to have a career like theirs and if so, why?

- What is appealing (or not) about what they do/did?

1.2 Why might it be good to consider a portfolio career?

A portfolio career is more than the definition above and it is more than juggling multiple jobs or careers simultaneously. I think that there are several key benefits:

- **Career autonomy** – a portfolio career allows you to exert control over your career and ultimately a large part of your life. Career autonomy is particularly difficult to achieve in a profession like medicine, especially as a junior hospital doctor. However, as a GP there is much more room for manoeuvre.
- **Multiple income streams** – portfolio careers can be a great way to generate several streams of income which may, eventually, contribute to better financial security and further career autonomy.
- **Variety** – you can experience immense career variety, gain the chance to learn new skills and develop existing ones further.
- **Reducing the chance of burnout** – medical students and doctors suffer from alarming rates of mental health issues throughout their careers. A portfolio career may be a 'protective factor', helping to reduce the likelihood of burnout or even stop it happening completely.

> When I was a trainee, I suffered from burnout so many times it ended up leaving me very frustrated and unfulfilled in both my personal and professional lives. I was trying to achieve what seemed impossible; I was trying to keep all my passions and interests alive but failing terribly. One by one my interests were discarded, like old clothes into a pile for a jumble sale, as I kept prioritising medicine above other non-medical interests I once enjoyed. My story is not unique; there are countless medics at various stages in their career feeling this way. You may even be one of them. On the other hand, a portfolio career is in itself a balancing act and so you must be careful not to try to do too much, which could lead to burnout...

Carving out your own portfolio career, created around your needs, skill set or lack thereof (which by the way does not have to stay the same for the duration of your working life!) ultimately helps us to become better doctors. This in turn enables us to serve our patients to the very best of our ability.

1.3 What challenges might you face when creating a portfolio career?

A portfolio career is not for everyone, and considerable thought should be given to some of the challenges that could arise:

- **Stigma of working part-time** – in medicine especially there can be a real stigma associated with working less than full-time. You might be seen by colleagues as not taking your job seriously enough or not being as committed as your peers. It may even be considered that you are not actually enjoying your career enough to want to do it full-time.
- **Financial commitments and responsibilities** – this can be particularly relevant early on in your career when you first take on significant rent or mortgage payments, coupled with repaying student loans. You may also have children and/or older relatives to care for. Reducing your GP hours to pursue other potentially less well-paid roles can obviously be seen as a risk, though as noted above, multiple income streams may give you greater security in the longer term.
- **How best to proceed** – many GPs have no clear idea or plan about how/when to start creating a portfolio career and this is compounded by limited structured information on the topic. Another reason may be lack of support and guidance in the form of mentorship.

1.4 Why are portfolio careers important now?

Portfolio careers have always been important for the reasons listed above (see *Section 1.2*). However, considering a portfolio career now is more important than ever as the NHS struggles to recruit and retain doctors in the UK. Despite rising numbers of students going to medical school, research shows that there has been a reduction in the number of fully qualified GPs (full-time equivalents) since 2015 and an increase in the number of GPs considering leaving the profession, with many looking to leave medicine entirely. Portfolio careers, as mentioned earlier, can help to reduce burnout and lead to happier and more fulfilled doctors, with a better work–life balance; such doctors are more likely to remain within the profession for longer.

In wider society there are many other factors that have meant portfolio careers are, now more than ever, being considered by many in different sectors worldwide, including primary care physicians. Such factors include:

- **Digitalisation** – with the growing use of technology across the board, engaging with and harnessing technology is now more important than ever to stay current and survive in the competitive job market. Individuals who recognise this are upskilling and finding ways to integrate and use technological advancements to broaden their prospects and improve their careers. Understanding how to code, create content, and use apps and novel platforms to improve efficiency in the NHS, are just some options that GPs may use to develop new opportunities and new income streams.

- **Collaborative and multi-generational working** – we are increasingly required to work with others, across generations and disciplines, across different time zones and cultures, and so have had to adjust to working remotely or virtually. The traditional hierarchy of management (in some sectors at least) has and will continue to become less important relative to the level and number of skills one has. Employers on the other hand continue to need the best employees, particularly those who are multi-faceted with broad skill sets. This means that employees may now be hired from anywhere in the world to help businesses stay current and profitable. As a UK-based GP, it is now easier than ever before to develop aspects of a portfolio career anywhere in the world by working remotely.

- **Career autonomy** – a portfolio career is one where the individual takes more control of how, when, where and for whom they work. In addition to the changes to the ways of working noted above, hybrid and flexible working provides more opportunities for the individual to take responsibility for their work and their career. For instance, as a GP there is a strong emphasis on self-directed learning and Continuing Professional Development (CPD) activities, either as mandatory e-learning or part of your e-portfolio. Taking responsibility for staying up to date is an integral part of working as a GP, and is even more important as a locum GP when you are not necessarily part of the practice team. Taking control of your learning provides the building blocks for developing your portfolio career as a GP (and makes the transition easier) because as a portfolio GP you will take control of other aspects such as your working schedule and the opportunities or jobs you decide to pursue. So, a portfolio career might be a natural transition and even inevitable part of future working life for many.

- **Covid-19 and innovation** – the pandemic accelerated how we use technology, especially within the NHS. It also brought about more of a 'forced' acceptance from many who were initially resistant to employing new technological methods. Individuals and companies have had to adapt and find innovative solutions to change that they never had to before, becoming more resilient in the process. The pandemic also allowed many people to realise that there are other options and other ways of working.

So now is the ideal time to consider additional or alternative career options for yourself; doing so is likely to be beneficial for you, the NHS and the patients we serve.

1.5 Traditional GP roles and the portfolio career

Traditionally there are three main ways GPs can work:

1. As a GP partner (also known as a GP contractor, a GP who is self-employed or a GP who holds a contract for services with NHS England, for example) – responsible for running a GP surgery, usually with other partners.
2. As a salaried or sessional GP who is employed by one or more practices, and works a set number of sessions per week.
3. As a locum GP (a GP who is self-employed or a GP with a contract for services) – historically considered as temporary GPs, but there are GPs who have longer-term locum positions.

GPs may also work in the following ways:

- As a GP with an extended role (previously known as a GP with a specialist interest, or GPwSI) – this role requires additional training such as completing a diploma. The role may be in a different setting, such as a community clinic, or offered outside of regular clinical duties in a GP surgery (for a set price or fee).
- As an out-of-hours GP – these GPs work outside of the usual core hours (typically covering 6.30pm – 8am during the weekdays, in addition to weekends and bank holidays). This type of working is usually associated with a higher salary than standard general practice rates.
- As a GP fellow – newly qualified GPs (within five years post CCT) can join a scheme to develop an interest in a variety of areas such

as a particular specialty (and become a GP with an extended role), leadership or education.

- The GP retention scheme – this is to support GPs with keeping their skills and knowledge up to date if they are unable to work a certain number of hours during the week.

A portfolio GP can work in any of the ways mentioned above as the 'foundation' block of their portfolio work. Of course, working as a locum GP offers the most flexibility, but salaried GPs working perhaps two to four sessions a week can use the remainder of their time to work on their other careers.

There are obviously advantages and disadvantages to working in the main ways above, and below is a summary of the features of each way of working.

Locum GP

- Usually self-employed, but locum GPs can also work through a limited company, a recruitment / locum agency and locum chambers (though this is uncommon).
- Typically earns more per session than a salaried GP and in some cases than a partner (with one session equivalent to one clinic or four hours of clinical work); can earn anywhere between £75 and £100 per hour, with the rate varying depending on the sector and location. Annual income could be £75 000–100 000 working full-time (and more than this if you are willing to work evenings and weekends). Some practices also include payments towards the NHS pension.
- Most flexible option, even when working a long-term post. Locum GPs can choose their working hours and patterns. No limit on leave, for example, unless specifically agreed otherwise with the practice. However, there may be some uncertainty around regular work and lack of employee rights and benefits, given that a locum GP is not an employed, permanent member of staff.

Salaried GP

- Employed by the practice so will have job security and employee entitlements, resulting in more stability than a locum GP.
- Usually earns between £9000 and £11 000 per session (may go up to £12 000). There is a minimum salary (advised by the Review Body on Doctors' and Dentists' Remuneration) if they

are working under the model salaried GP contract from the BMA which, at the time of writing, is £58 808 to £88 744. There can be a variation in pay across the UK; however, salary can be negotiated. Some things to consider when negotiating would be experience and additional skills, e.g. a cardiology diploma.

- Limited flexibility because there will be a set number of annual and study leave days in addition to fixed sessions at the practice (often including a minimum number to commit to). Most salaried GPs are not expected to work outside the hours of 8am – 6.30pm, although in reality most probably will, even though doing so will not affect pay. Practices providing out-of-hours services will require salaried GPs to work beyond core hours.

GP partner

- Also known as a GP contractor, they are self-employed, which may offer more stability because a partnership is usually a longer-term commitment.
- Pay after expenses is deducted from the practice income; this pay is called 'drawings' or profits. There are other factors to consider such as working capital and employees' pensions, in addition to the partner's own pension. GP partners working full-time typically earn between £100 000 and £140 000 per annum, depending in part on the location they are working in. Working together in a partnership has the advantage of sharing the responsibility of managing a practice. However, partners may have to 'buy in' to the practice and are personally liable for any financial issues.

1.6 How this book can help you

There is very little in the way of career support for medics, especially for those just starting out in their careers – this was certainly true for me. Some progress has been made, but there still seems to be insufficient support and advice for junior doctors in particular.

In my time as a GP trainee there was very little in the way of formal career support, during either one-to-one sessions with my trainer or group sessions with other trainees – any support we did receive was usually in the form of informal conversations and questions asked over lunch (if time!). Research about what opportunities are available has to be done largely in your own time, by speaking to others (within and outside of the medical profession), attending courses and conferences and completing online learning. There remains very little in the way of information pertaining to portfolio careers for doctors, which is where this book comes in!

This book will provide you with a background to portfolio careers within medicine, as well as show you what is possible through the career stories of the incredible GPs showcased in this book. If you're interested in creating a portfolio career but have no idea where to begin, then this book will act as a starting point for you on your journey. You may already have an idea or be working on a portfolio career but want to learn more and explore other avenues and opportunities; if so, then you can use this book to help you find more clarity and refine your ideas. Please feel free to skip ahead to *Chapter 6* for more information about what is possible to achieve, but do take some time to read the whole book, which is designed to help you create a portfolio career step by step:

- *Chapter 2* – describes the basic principles of career development, and how to develop a deeper understanding of exactly who you are, and takes into consideration wider factors that can affect you and the development of your portfolio career.
- *Chapter 3* – here you will learn what career success means to you and how you can achieve it.
- *Chapter 4* – shows practical applications of what you have learnt in previous chapters; how you can categorise your portfolio activities, taking into consideration financial and legal implications, time management, balancing your workload and how to set goals to stay on track to creating a successful portfolio career tailored to you.
- *Chapter 5* – explains why it is important to continuously evaluate your career and how you can go about doing this – the process is never complete!
- *Chapter 6* – looks at the work of a number of GPs who have created portfolio careers they are really happy with; you can use them as inspiration and examples of what is possible.

Whether you are just starting out in general practice, starting to think about a move to a portfolio career, and wanting to upgrade your current portfolio, the book provides lots of practical advice for you to create the career most suited to you and, most importantly, one that you are excited to develop.

Chapter 2:
Planning for a portfolio career

By the end of this chapter you should be able to:

- Feel that you have developed a deeper understanding of who you are and where you fit within the wider constructs of society
- Apply the basic principles of career development theory to your own emerging portfolio career.

Chapter 1 provided a background to portfolio careers and how they fit into our ever-evolving society. Now we can begin looking at the steps you need to take to create your own portfolio career.

2.1 **The importance of career development in medicine**

One of the primary aims of medical schools is to prepare students for the clinical aspects of working life as a doctor, and medical schools focus (and quite rightly so) on the requirements of the GMC's *Good Medical Practice*. However, working as a doctor also requires non-clinical knowledge and skills, such as:

- creating a medical CV and career portfolio
- financial literacy
- understanding employee contracts and rights
- leadership and managerial skills.

These may not always be gained during your time at medical school, even if you have participated in a wide variety of extracurricular activities. Medical schools do try to support students with career development, but the quality of this support varies across medical schools. This might be due to lack of adequate mentors, lack of sufficient time to develop non-clinical skills, and the stigma associated with some topics, such as mental health and financial literacy.

You might think that if you don't learn the non-clinical knowledge and skills whilst at medical school, then surely you would once you start working life as a doctor?

Ultimately this lack of knowledge and missing non-clinical skill set may lead to reduced fulfilment with your career, poor mental health, financial difficulties and, at its worst, to you considering leaving the profession. As medics most of us have experienced, first-hand, the problematic systems and structures in place that can significantly affect our career development. But now let's look at other factors (internal factors pertaining to you) that can influence your career and how they might manifest over time.

2.2 Are you ready for a portfolio career?

Before considering planning (or re-planning) your career, you might want to take a moment and consider whether you are really ready to begin this journey (we will go through career planning readiness in more detail in *Section 3.3*).

Whilst we work through *Section 2.3*, think carefully about:

- whether a change in your career (even a small one) is the right choice *now*
- what is motivating you to consider a portfolio career
- whether you are looking to refine your career, or wanting to take it in a completely new direction.

2.3 The first steps to developing your career

First things first: before you can begin creating your portfolio career, you need to analyse exactly who you are. To help you do this, it is worth being aware of four key career development theories:

- Parsons' (1909) trait factor theory. This theory is also known as the talent-matching or matching theory; a person aims to understand their own personality traits, abilities and interests and then seeks to match them against the requirements of different jobs.
- Ginzberg *et al.*'s 1951 theory of occupational choice; a 'developmental theory'. Ginzberg *et al.* thought about occupational choice evolving through various stages or periods in one's life.

- Super, in his 1953 career development theory (also a 'developmental' theory), developed Ginzberg's work, identifying limitations which helped in formulating a theory including various career development stages and tasks. His future work involved a more holistic approach than Ginzberg's, with its foundations in systemic thinking.
- Systems theory: a more contemporary view of career development. This theory considers multiple factors or systems in relation to career development; they are integrated to such an extent that they cannot be separated.

What do these career development theories have to do with creating my portfolio career?

Reviewing theories such as these exposes you to different ways of thinking and therefore to the possibilities that could be open to you. They can be used to help you learn more about yourself and your environment, and to provide you with the clarity needed to build strong foundations for your own career. The rest of this chapter will help you to put the theories into practice.

So, what exactly is career development?

It can be defined as an ongoing process of understanding yourself and the world around you, and using that to inform your choices and therefore career trajectory (which includes a collection of your jobs and/or vocations).

Career development is a lifelong journey encompassing self-discovery, transition and change. Some people meticulously plan their career and others act more impulsively, grabbing opportunities and saying 'yes' to various experiences that come their way. Others may use a combination of the two; I have certainly used a combination of planning and exploring new opportunities or experimenting (based on my interests) during my career (see *Example 2.1*).

Example 2.1

Whilst on The Emerging Women Leaders course at University College London, I had the opportunity to hear from some extraordinary women. Many of the leaders I listened to agreed that their career (and career success) had been a combination of planned and in some cases largely unplanned, seemingly serendipitous events.

They also highlighted additional pertinent points:

- Career development does not have to be a strategic, meticulously planned process:
  - saying 'yes' to more opportunities can lead you to new and exciting pathways and career success
  - sometimes you have to create opportunities for yourself and set an example.
- Career development is complex and impacted by many factors such as family, social circumstances, personality traits and life events.
- Their successful careers were also due to advice from mentors.
- Having multiple mentors (who have different skill sets and connections) is crucial to career success and personal development.
- Look out for advocates. These are individuals who will go the extra mile to help you; speaking positively about you to others and putting you forward for opportunities (also known as sponsorship, which we will discuss later; see *Section 3.6*). Consider those who you may not initially think would necessarily want to or be able to help you.

Now, let's see how we can put the theories outlined above into practice. The following section explains how the career development theories are useful for you to critically evaluate and use when developing your own career.

2.4 The importance of assessing your interests, skills, qualities and achievements

You may have applied to medical school because you felt working as a doctor was more than a job, it was a vocation; I personally had (and still have) that view. Frank Parsons held similar views. He was the American academic who created the talent-matching theory, also known as the matching theory or the trait factor theory.

To choose the right career, according to the talent-matching theory, you should fully understand yourself, including your personal abilities and interests, and the requirements of the job market. Based on this information you should ideally find a 'match' which should (hopefully) be the right choice for you. This sounds easy to do in principle; however, you may need to consider changes to your personal development, your circumstances, and changes within the job market itself. Finally, you might find that you 'match' to multiple careers instead of just one 'right' one. Perhaps you could consider undertaking this 'matching' process several times throughout your career?

In the sections which follow, there are a few questions you can use to get to know yourself that little bit better. Try to answer the questions as fully as possible.

2.4.1 Interests

What are you interested in and what are your preferences?

For example, do you enjoy writing? If so, medical or opinion-based articles? Personally, although I have *had* to write factual pieces during medical school and training, I *prefer* writing opinion-based articles and poetry because I find them therapeutic. This is not to say I am not interested in the former, but I have recognised as I have developed that I prefer to write more creatively and have therefore pursued this avenue both as a hobby and career.

Note down your interests below *(I've added a few examples to get you started)*:

Art – painting, sculpting

Education

Paediatrics

Now go through your list above and rank your top ten interests.

- Can you 'match' any of your interests with any jobs you know of?
- Do any of these matches interest you as potential careers?
  - if so, what factors could influence your decision to pursue this career path now or in the future?
  - for example, might it be too expensive to start right now? If considering a career in, say, occupational health and aiming to complete the diploma, the costs for the initial two-week course, examination and any revision books / course could reach £3000.

Repeat your top 10 interests below and add matching jobs
(I've added an example to get you started):

Interest	Possible job	Why is / isn't this an option?
Education	Medical school lecturer	No experience

2.4.2 Achievements

What are your achievements?

Which of your achievements might support any of the job options identified above?

Examples include *recorded* achievements during your career. Using the writing example from above:

- Do you have any journal publications? If so, what are they? What was your role in the publication and why did you have this role?
- Do you have any blog pieces you've written for credible organisations and companies?

Note your achievements below *(I've added a few examples to get you started)*:

Qualifications   Medical degree; intercalated BSc

Prizes   At medical school but also for extracurricular activities

Next steps:

List the achievements you are most proud of and note down why, but also be honest and add whether there are things that you can do to improve:

Achievement   Why are you proud of this? Can you improve further?

2.4.3 Skills and qualities

What skills and qualities do you have?

Are you quite a patient person, and do you have high levels of self-discipline when it comes to carrying out tasks? Are you a good communicator? Do you pride yourself on being very organised or able to delegate tasks to others appropriately? Personally, I believe I am a good written and verbal communicator; however, there is still much room for improvement!

Note down your skills and qualities below (*I've added a few examples to get you started*):

Time management

Resilience

Problem solving

The next step is to think especially about the skills you used most to gain your achievements. List your achievements from earlier, in order of importance (from 1 to 10, for example) and then assign the skills required for each one. This may well then demonstrate a trend of the skills you use most to achieve.

Note your achievements in order of importance and then assign a skill and/or quality to each one (*I've added a couple of examples to get you started*), but also note any skills that you think could be improved:

Qualifications   Hard working

Prizes   Competitive

Now compare your original list of skills and qualities with those that you have ascribed to your achievements – which skills do you utilise the most and which do you not use enough? How can you improve this balance? For example, perhaps you are terrible at organising your weekly tasks, which then leads you to procrastinate. On the other hand, you are great at researching new technologies and platforms. Maybe you can use your excellent research skills to look for the best artificial intelligence (AI) tools or virtual assistants that might help improve your organisation.

2.4.4 Values and beliefs

What are the principles you live by and what do you believe to be true about yourself?

Our values are the standards or principles by which we live. Examples include honesty and loyalty.

Our beliefs are what we believe to be true, which can be assumptions about the world around us. Examples are: (self) I am confident and capable of making good decisions; (others / the world) the world is a cruel place to live in. Understanding what values and beliefs you hold about yourself and the world will help ensure you are on the path that aligns with what you truly believe in.

Take a moment to list your core values and beliefs here:

Values   Beliefs

You should now have more of an in-depth understanding of yourself, comprising crucial aspects of who you are and what you believe in (your values, beliefs, strengths, weaknesses and so on). You might find it useful to use the template below to create a short summary of what you have uncovered.

In *Chapter 4* we will then use this information to help create an actual portfolio of activities, specific to you, that will help you in creating your portfolio career.

Top 3 achievements

1.

2.

3.

Top 3 interests

1.

2.

3.

Top 3 skills and qualities

1.

2.

3.

Top 3 values and beliefs

1.

2.

3.

2.5 Understanding how time and the wider environment impact your career

According to Ginzberg and Super (see *Section 2.3* if you need a reminder of their theories) there are other factors to think about as you consider how to develop your portfolio career. We will now look at the following factors that Ginzberg highlighted in his theory of occupational choice.

Careers can take a long time to develop

You might see this in your own journey so far. As a GP it has taken me:

- six years of medical school training (including intercalation)
- two years of foundation training
- one gap year (feeling very confused about my career)
- three years of GP training and (at the time of writing) four years working as a GP (and I am still trying to find my feet!).

Since qualifying I have also undertaken various locum and salaried opportunities, including remote and face-to-face roles.

Careers can be difficult to reverse out of

Due to the significant investments of time (as above) and money, in addition to personal changes, we can sometimes feel 'stuck' in an unfulfilling career.

Careers are often a compromise

They can be a compromise based on interests, values, capacities and opportunities. But you need to consider whether your current career is an acceptable compromise or is one-sided. How can you make it more balanced if it isn't currently?

A career may be impacted by life stages / personal development which can alter outlook

Your career development alters at various stages and may begin as early as childhood. As a child you may have felt the possibilities were endless, but of course you had no clear or realistic plan about how to achieve your career goals and whether the careers you considered really suited your personality, skills and capabilities.

> For me personally, when I decided I wanted to become a doctor at the age of four, I had no idea if this was achievable or even suited who I was as a person. As I matured, my perspective shifted to a more realistic outlook on my career choices. This was based on my growing interests, capacities, values and beliefs. Finally, as I qualified, I had a much deeper understanding of who I was, the real-life challenges in medicine, and the interaction between myself and work. As time has progressed I have refined (and continue to refine) my career choices, which includes focusing on the essential requirements (for example, needing to gain postgraduate qualifications) required for my career success.

Before moving on to the final theory ('systems theory'), let's look at some additional key takeaways from Super, who further developed Ginzberg's work:

- We are all unique, with different interests and abilities. *You should not compare your career to someone else's!*
- Everyone has the potential to be successful in multiple careers. *If you do not feel successful, what can you do to change this? Do you believe you have potential? If so, what could be holding you back? Could it be you or is it the systems around you?*

- Career development is not only based on your unique set of abilities, skills and personality. It can be supported by having access to relevant opportunities. *Were there opportunities you feel you may have missed or not had access to? Why do you think this was? How do you think this has affected your career pattern, i.e. the nature and frequency of your permanent and/or temporary jobs?*
- You have specific patterns of abilities and interests that are well suited to certain occupations. These patterns help to determine if you are likely to choose a particular occupation and, more importantly, stay and be happy in that occupation. *Do you think your identified skills and interests are well suited to your current career? If not, why not? How could you find out which careers they could be better suited to?*
- Individuals (especially children and adolescents) identify with other people, such as their parents and teachers, and this can impact on career development. *Can you remember this far back? Did you identify with anyone when you were growing up and why? Has this changed now?*
- During the process of developing your career, you will progress through different life stages, but it is important to stay open-minded. You may be in the process of exploring different careers and/or more firmly establishing existing ones. For example, you might be refining your clinical skills as a GP but exploring other options such as performing minor surgeries or aesthetic procedures. *What stage are you at? Do you want to be there? What can you do to progress to another stage?*
- The only way you will develop your career is by engaging with the outside world. You need to get yourself 'out there'. Say 'yes' to opportunities, think about taking small risks and trying new things. *Have you tried applying for a role that you may have felt slightly underqualified for?*

> *I applied for a role as a course lead and ended up being offered a senior lecturer role; this could then lead to other opportunities such as a course lead on another programme.*

- Career development is a continuous process of adjustment; over time people (including their career preferences) and their environment (including their working environments) change. This affects how people view themselves (i.e. the self-concept):
  - *Who are you? How do you see yourself and why? What do you feel your identity is?*

- *What changes have you noticed about yourself over the years and why do you think these changes have come about?*
- *What changes might you foresee as you develop in skill set, experience and age?*

Of course, whilst helpful, there are limitations with any theoretical perspective and it is important to be mindful of this. The statements and questions above are designed to get you *thinking*.

The systems theory framework considers multiple factors or systems in relation to career development. These systems comprise, at their most basic:

- The individual (intrapersonal components such as personality, the self-concept, gender, age, ethnicity)
- Society and the wider environment (the individual's family, peers, education, work, globalisation, socioeconomic status and geographical location).

There is also an acknowledgment of how these systems are affected by time and serendipity.

So far, although we have considered the wider environment, the *main* focus has been more on you as a person – *your* personality, *your* skills and qualities, *your* interests, *your* passions and hobbies. However, you do not exist in isolation. We all exist within wider ever-changing circumstances that ultimately affect our choices when carving out our careers.

Take some time to think about other factors that have affected (and will affect) your career development.

- *List three ways your career choices have been impacted by:*
  - Your family and your peers / your ethnicity / your education history / your finances
  - The geographical location of where you have to (or have had to) work
  - The political environment

- *Which of the factors above are most important and hence will have a greater impact on your future career choices?*
- *How will the factors above affect your career in the future?*

Note which factors have affected your career choices so far (past and present) and then consider which may impact on your career in the future:

Factors	Past	Present	Future
Family: having a child	changed ways of working, i.e. working remotely	working more face-to-face, with remote to supplement as child is older	will increase hours as child reaches school age but not back to full-time so can spend more time with family.

- Does anything bother you about the above factors and if so, can you do anything to change this?

> *For example:* I am worried about how my career will be impacted if I expand my family, i.e. have a second child. Looking for other streams of income / expanding my skill set / asking for help from my employer, colleagues and family could help.

This is just the beginning; in *Chapter 4* we will use all of this valuable information about you and your environment to create your very own portfolio career.

I hope this chapter has provided you with a *starting point* of how you can get to know yourself better.

Learning about who you are is a crucial step in creating a portfolio career and cannot be neglected. From experience and research,

I think many people simply dive into choosing a career without ever really analysing themselves and establishing if they would be well-suited to the patterns of abilities required for that occupation.

You have used key elements from various career development theories to draw out crucial thoughts regarding who you are, how you relate to the world around you and what you truly want for your career. You have started applying this information in a practical way, which will help you turn your ideas into reality.

Even if you are certain you want to create a portfolio career, I think at this point it is too early to decide if you are truly ready. I also think it is too early at this point, from what we have covered, to know what your ideal portfolio career would look like. What I would say is that you have probably learnt lots more about yourself. You may also have recognised that your choices have been influenced significantly by your immediate and wider environment more than you may have realised before. So, hold onto this valuable information and let's continue to build on this as we progress through to the next chapter.

Chapter summary

- Career development is a complex, ongoing process which is influenced by both internal factors (you) and external factors (the environment).
- The starting point to developing a portfolio career is to fully understand who you are and how you have changed (and will change in the future) – the boxes you completed at the end of *Section 2.4* help with this.
- Understanding yourself, your environment and the resulting interaction is fundamental to creating a strong foundation for your career development.
- Career development theories enable you to explore different perspectives and help you begin to apply key principles to your own career, helping you decide in which direction to go.

Chapter 3:
Setting yourself up for career success

By the end of this chapter you should be able to:

- Describe what career success is, what it means to you and how you can achieve success in your own career
- List the four key predictors of career success and start thinking about how these can be applied to your own career
- Utilise crucial self-help aids that will be essential for successful career planning and development.

In this first section, we will look at what career success is, what it means to you and the key predictors of career success (the factors influencing your level of success).

3.1 Defining what career success looks like to you

What we are trying to answer, deep down, is how can we create a successful career(s) that ultimately, we are truly happy with? The fact that you picked up this book means that there is something you're looking for, something you haven't yet discovered in your current career.

Many of us might not be finding complete fulfilment with one career, route or pathway. As we have seen this could be for a few reasons.

- For one, we are all different individuals with a variety of interests, skills and qualities that some of us want to actively improve upon and nurture. We might be frustrated that we are unable to pursue other interests or develop different skills in the way that we want or as quickly as we would like.

- We may not be completely happy with the wider systems and structures in place, which then leads to frustrations in a career we may have once been (perhaps seemingly) satisfied with. This could be due to a lack of support during training, post Certificate of Completion of Training (CCT) or a lack of funding and financial assistance from the government and/or perceived mismanagement of said funds.

- We might feel torn because there are some aspects of this career we particularly enjoy and some that we don't.

So, a compromise of working part-time or with less responsibility (a locum or part-time salaried GP instead of a partner) allows us to take a step back to create time to step up in other, hopefully more enjoyable and freeing roles or ways of working.

> So, how can we go about creating a successful career? Is this **really** possible, especially when we have families and financial commitments to consider?

If you asked two people to define career success, you might get very different answers! However, one thing I have realised from speaking to many medics of various generations (and of course my own perspective) is that career success is much more than seniority and financial reward. Of course, money is important for obvious reasons, but how much money you earn does not necessarily define how successful you are or feel you are. Other factors such as personal satisfaction, fulfilment, achievement, opportunities, and simply enjoying your career are also important reasons as to why people feel they are successful (or unsuccessful) on their career path.

So, whilst there may not be a 'one size fits all' approach, there are some important points to consider in this chapter which will hopefully help you create a successful career, tailored to you.

3.1.1   What is career success?

Since we are unique, and our experiences are not the same, our definitions of career success will vary. In short, career success is a combination of positive outcomes related to work; outcomes which are both work-related and psychological.

Career success can be broadly divided into objective (or extrinsic) and subjective (or intrinsic) factors:

- Objective factors include salary and promotions which can lead others to think a person is successful, when perhaps the individual in question may not agree
- Subjective factors include job satisfaction, and they represent the individual's perception of their success.

This is why you should not compare yourself to others and how they appear to be doing.

Working out what success means to you

- Do you currently feel satisfied in your job and if not, why not?

- What can you do to improve this?

- Can it be improved?

By understanding what success means to you, what motivates you and what doesn't, you will (hopefully) be able to shape a career that will be both enjoyable and exciting, withstanding the test of time and wider external influences.

3.2 How can you achieve career success?

There are four main steps to follow in your quest for success:

- **Understanding:** which types of career success are important to you and why?
- **Recognising:** the journey towards career success requires mobility
- **Appreciating:** there are key predictors of career success
- **Maximising:** the key predictors of career success.

We will now work through each of these steps in order.

3.2.1 Understanding: which types of career success are important to you and why?

As mentioned above, there are two forms of success: objective (extrinsic) and subjective (intrinsic). An important step when creating your portfolio career is to decide which forms of success are most important to you (or perhaps they are all equally important?). This will help you with current and future choices regarding the direction of your career and which opportunities to say 'yes' and 'no' to. We all measure our success through our salary, promotions, hierarchy and, of course, job satisfaction.

However, at times we might prioritise job satisfaction over pay, or vice versa. For me, the financial reward is of course important, but I could not work as a GP, writer, lecturer and so on if I did not personally enjoy what I was doing and gain a non-monetary reward. Take a minute to think about what is most important to you at the moment by completing the box below.

Find out what type of success is important to you

- Is objective or subjective success more important to you and why?

....

....

- Which factors are most important? Rank your top three.

....

....

....

- Could you compromise on one or more of them and still view yourself as successful?

....

....

3.2.2 Recognising: the journey towards career success requires mobility

There are three forms of mobility: upward, sponsored and contest mobility.

Upward mobility describes how those higher up a hierarchical system are seen as more successful, and so movement up this theoretical hierarchical ladder indicates success. This can be seen in medical students (especially those from less privileged backgrounds) graduating to become doctors and then moving up in seniority as they progress in their careers. Despite starting lower down the hierarchical ladder, they have climbed to the top and this is seen as a significant indicator of career success to themselves and to those around them.

Sponsored mobility is essentially when a powerful or elite individual or organisation supports someone (usually someone who has demonstrated significant potential such as a 'future leader') so that they can achieve career progression and more success.

Contest mobility is when an individual's career success is dependent solely on their own individual efforts. This view assumes that the playing field is level for everyone. Usually in life, as you can imagine (or have experienced!), a combination of both sponsored and contest mobility exists. Using the above example of medical school – upward mobility is therefore influenced by both sponsored mobility (it helps if you have connections to get into medical school) and contest mobility (you also need a significant level of individual effort).

3.2.3 Appreciating: there are key predictors of career success

Understanding the key predictors of career success can help you carve out your career and achieve the level of success you desire. Looking at what has happened in your past (and what can be done differently going forward) will help you make the necessary choices and right decisions for your uniquely designed career.

The four key predictors of success are as follows:

- **Human capital** – an individual's inherent abilities which are gradually improved on through various activities and experiences. This predictor includes your educational level, working history (where you have worked and for how long) and your *social capital* (your network of contacts). Human capital is discussed in more detail in *Section 3.3*, and social capital in *Section 3.5*.
- **Organisational sponsorship** – the support provided by an organisation to enhance your career. This includes career sponsorship (support from senior colleagues), training and resources (the number of resources you have access to is usually related somewhat to the size of the organisation you work for). This is covered in more detail in *Section 3.6*.
- **Socio-demographic status** – your gender, race, age and marital status (covered later in this section).

- **Stable individual differences** – the 'Big Five' personality traits: neuroticism, conscientiousness, extroversion, agreeableness, and openness to experience (covered below).

So, success is a combination of your own effort (hard work, determination – contest mobility) and help from other, more senior people around you (which could be through informal / formal mentoring activities – sponsored mobility). Furthermore, to be successful it is important to set yourself apart from the competition (we are competing for jobs, higher pay and so on), promote yourself (perhaps via effective personal branding) and remain positive (because there will be ups and downs).

Here are a few questions to ask yourself:

- How can you set yourself apart from the competition? Be specific: what activities can you do to enhance your career and do what no one else is doing?

- How can you promote yourself in a way that might get the right people (employers) to notice you?

- Are you a naturally positive person? If you're not, what techniques could you employ to ensure you are more positive?

Of the four predictors, human capital and organisational sponsorship are the most important for the purpose of this book and so they will be covered in much more detail in subsequent sections. But here I'll briefly provide you with important points to consider regarding the impact of personality and socio-demographic factors on career success.

Stable individual differences (the impact of personality)

The type of personality you have is closely linked to **subjective** career success.

> How much your organisation helps you is also closely linked to subjective career success.

If you are more 'extroverted', less 'neurotic' or less 'agreeable', you may be more satisfied with your career.

> Furthermore, being more of an extrovert may lead to better pay and more promotions.

- Research has shown that being extroverted is beneficial regardless of where you work (for example, it does not matter if your job requires having good social skills or not). This may be because extroverted individuals prefer being social (and are presumed to have good social or interpersonal skills), they may make others become more aware of their presence and influence, and this in turn may lead to further development of their social skills (and social networks).

Finally, being more positive and ready to make changes when not happy are also important components in achieving subjective success.

Overall, possessing the personality characteristics of an extroverted individual seems to lead to greater subjective (and objective) success.

Regarding personality characteristics

If you are not naturally extroverted, is there anything you can do when interacting with others or with organisations which could potentially help improve your baseline level of success?

You may not agree completely with the Big Five assessment, but it can be a useful tool to help you reflect on your own personality type and how this might impact your level of success. I have taken the assessment and there were certainly aspects I agreed with (and some that I did not!). You might also be interested in the three updated versions of the initial personality inventory by Costa and McCrae; I preferred the shorter version with sixty items (NEO-FFI) (you can find this in *Appendix 1: Further reading*).

Socio-demographic status

*Socio-demographic status may have more bearing on **objective** career success.*

> Human capital and work experience have been shown to impact both subjective and objective career success, but they also have more bearing on objective success.

- A typical example of how socio-demographic status impacts on objective career success is when some organisations perceive that men are more valuable than women because men take fewer career breaks (women may have breaks for maternity leave, and women are more likely to work part-time to look after children). This is backed up by research which shows that women and ethnic minorities earn lower wages than their respective counterparts. The *Mend the Gap* report (2020) demonstrates that a gender pay gap remains even after accounting for variations in working hours: for hospital doctors (18.9%), GPs (15.3%) and clinical academics (11.9%).

Whilst it might be hard to overcome stereotypes or perceptions such as for gender, being aware of perceptions can help you to challenge these stereotypes and modify your behaviour, including your own self-perception.

- For example, research among STEM (Science, Technology, Engineering and Mathematics) graduates has shown that a 'confidence gap' exists (women tend to have less confidence or self-efficacy than men), and this is an important reason for the difference between men's and women's salaries. Furthermore, other research demonstrates that women are less likely to take risks, negotiate and be competitive compared to men. Women appear to have fewer opportunities to negotiate (for a variety of possible reasons) but when they do, they do not appear to perform less well than men, resulting in better wage outcomes.

If this sounds like you, what could you do to change this? Could you think about potentially negotiating your salary when starting a new job, or what about asking for a salary uplift in your current one? This is just one example but hopefully it gives you some food for thought.

3.2.4 Maximising: the key predictors of career success

It is not enough to simply 'appreciate' that there are four key predictors of career success. You must put them into practice and use them to your advantage. Think about what we have covered so far – how can you start learning about your personality type and adjusting necessary aspects to maximise your chance of success? How can you be more aware of how your socio-demographic status (such as your gender and ethnicity) impacts your level of career success and what can you do to counteract this?

Through further exploration of the two key predictors (human capital and organisational sponsorship) in the following sections, we will look at how you can fully utilise the key predictors, creating a clear advantage for yourself.

> **Section summary**
> - Career success can be viewed both objectively and subjectively; it is usually a combination of the two. Objective (or extrinsic) career success includes how much you earn, while subjective (or intrinsic) career success is how satisfied you feel in your career.
> - People place different weighting on the types of success. Now is the time for you to reflect on how you define career success and how much emphasis you place on subjective and objective aspects. You can use the box below to help.
> - There are four key predictors of career success: human capital, organisational sponsorship, socio-demographic status and stable individual differences.
> - Remember that career success is also affected by a combination of contest and sponsored mobility.

Practical exercise – defining success

How do you define career success?

Important subjective factors

Important objective factors

The rest of this chapter will take a closer look at two of the four key predictors (human capital and organisational sponsorship) because these are the two areas where you have the greatest ability to make changes. We will focus on how you can maximise the various elements to create a successful career.

3.3 How to assess your qualifications and work experience

Human capital, broadly speaking, encompasses the following:

- Your baseline education level, obtaining additional qualifications, **evaluating work experience to date and gaining valuable work experiences in the future** (described in this section)
- Career planning (including self-help aids); covered in *Section 3.4*
- Social capital – building connections and gaining (and exchanging) resources; covered fully in *Section 3.5*.

At all times while creating your portfolio career it is important to consider how you can bring these elements together *practically*.

You might want to create a combination of employed, self-employed or freelance roles in your career. Or you may want to solely work as employee in two or three part-time roles; perhaps you feel being employed is the best option for you if you do not like the unpredictability of working as a freelancer. You want to know you have a steady income stream and secure work all year round, but simultaneously you'd like to have variety in your working week. If this is the case, you should concentrate on your potential *employer's perspective* and how you can enhance your job prospects to ensure you secure these roles. So, concentrating on improving your human capital would make the most sense, right?

On the other hand, perhaps you want to have more creative freedom and undertake predominantly or only freelance roles, or you want to start your own limited company and become self-employed. Let's say you want to specialise in delivering educational courses and training activities for corporate companies. You would therefore focus on your *client's perspective* and why they should hire you to train their employees or clients. But the approach is similar: you would focus on improving your human capital.

So, how can you do this?

3.3.1 Assessing your baseline education level and obtaining additional qualifications

Whilst education level is important in human capital theory, for obvious reasons as medical professionals our starting point is completion of training. Therefore, we will be focusing on postgraduate qualifications to see why obtaining these can benefit your career.

According to human capital theory, and as you have (hopefully) demonstrated by working through the early part of this book, you have many skills, qualities and abilities. Through your education, medical training and work experience you will have improved upon these and gained new ones too. So, theoretically, your worth to employers (and/or clients) should have increased, as should your level of career success and potentially your income. This assumption relies on this information being shared with your employer, or potential employer; they could access your human capital through websites where you can post your CV so employers can find you, social media networks such as LinkedIn, and speaking to others about your experience and qualifications.

As an example, let's say you have additional qualifications such as a diploma in cardiology and a Postgraduate Certificate in Medical

Education (PGCE). You have been working as a GP for ten years
and are currently a GP with an extended role at a practice. Here are
some things your employer would have made a note of:

- The necessary qualifications (MRCGP) and the basic required
  competences and skills (supported by your referees) for the job
- Additional qualifications that could be an advantage to the
  practice – postgraduate certificate and diploma (teaching roles,
  additional clinics)
- Your experience and length of time working as a GP – ten years
  as a GP would indicate an experienced GP, as would the variety
  of places you have worked.

According to signalling theory your additional qualifications and
length of experience would have been a 'signal' about your levels of
productivity at work. This signal would probably have culminated
in the employer seriously considering you for the role, in addition to
potentially offering a higher rate of pay per session; your significant
experience and additional qualifications (which should lead to
better outcomes for the practice) provide you with the 'leverage' to
attempt to negotiate your salary.

So, to summarise, gaining an additional qualification(s) results in:

- *Accumulating more human capital* – you will have more than the
  baseline MRCGP which all GP trainees are required to obtain, and
  probably more work experience
- *A positive signal* to your future employer (or client you want to
  work with)
- *Possibly more pay* (relative to someone who does not have that
  qualification).

Example 3.1 – How additional qualifications help

I believe I was offered a role as a lecturer at Ulster University (for
their Advanced General Medical Practice programme) because of
my qualifications, which included my intercalated BSc, professional
experience, working as a GP and being registered as a PLAB examiner
with the GMC (this was relevant to the new course the college wanted
to create). So, although I did not have a postgraduate qualification in
education, I had several other factors working in my favour.

However, having worked in the role I realised that developing a
deeper understanding of education would be beneficial. Furthermore,
some employers in this area categorise a postgraduate qualification
such as a PGCE as a minimum to apply for a post as a lecturer or MSc

programme lead. I have seen this first-hand in job applications I have viewed and applied for – and the lack of such an additional qualification may have been one of the reasons I was not offered these jobs. I did, however, gain lots of useful experience, such as learning how to create an MSc programme from scratch, which I felt future employers would find useful. I believe that it is this experience that has helped me secure my role as a senior lecturer for the Physician Associate (PA) programme at the University of East London.

Your thoughts on additional qualifications

• Have you considered additional qualifications? If so, which ones and why?

• How might you go about obtaining those and when might be a good time to do so?

• Is there anyone you can speak to about this?

3.3.2 Work experience past and future

I'd like to make two main points regarding work experience:

• I want you to realise that you have gained lots of transferable skills that can easily help you transition into another career or create a great portfolio career.
• Ensuring you have work experience in areas of interest is crucial, but equally you can learn something from all work experience you undertake.

Evaluate your previous and current work experiences

Evaluating your previous and current work experiences (even if predominantly in a clinical capacity) will help you determine the skills, especially the **transferable skills**, you have gained.

Skills such as leadership can be used in other clinical and non-clinical roles which can then translate into success in other aspects of your portfolio career.

Think about your transferable skills

List **three** transferable skills you have gained throughout your working history, for example, Problem-solving skills:

Clinically – there are always challenging problems to solve such as prescribing in an elderly patient with several co-morbidities, drug allergies and polypharmacy. This can be transferred to a career in the pharmaceutical industry (because...)

Personal life – trying to solve day-to-day problems that arise in relationships at home, or issues at school. This can be transferred (because...)

Moreover, if you have worked internationally, this could also be beneficial because it will have opened you up to new cultures, languages, and ways of working.

It might be worth reviewing job descriptions for previous jobs you have had and seeing how this truly correlated with your day-to-day work and what you gained (or did not gain) as a result.

Job descriptions vs. day-to-day working

List **two** jobs you have previously worked in, and for each, describe what you thought you had to do / were asked to do based on the job description, and what you had to do day-to-day, *for example,* working as a foundation year one doctor on an elderly care ward

What I thought I had to do	What I really had to do	What did I gain overall?
Primarily clinical work, assessing and managing patients	Predominantly administrative work such as writing discharge summaries, re-writing drug charts, requesting investigations as advised by senior colleagues	Improved communication skills, e.g. speaking to relatives and patients about end-of-life care

Improved clinical skills, e.g. blood taking, cannulation, catheterisation

The ability to work independently and find necessary information quickly, e.g. by speaking to a pharmacist, consulting the BNF and relevant guidelines |

- What work experiences have you had on your journey?

- Have you had any work experiences (including voluntary roles) abroad?

- Which experiences were good and perhaps not so good and why?

- Do you feel your job description reflects your current role(s) and if not, why not?

- If you did **not** gain the experience you were hoping for, what could you do going forward to change this?

It is usual to note the *length of time* you have worked for an organisation on your CV – typically each job and the time you undertook it for should be listed. The length of time you have worked somewhere, and hence your experience, can often affect your future job prospects. For example, having very short roles at

Example 3.2 – All your experiences can still be useful

As a portfolio GP, I have many roles listed on my CV and, when applying for jobs over the years, several employers have asked how I can manage all the roles. Their concern is that I cannot focus sufficiently on so many roles, which may affect my ability to undertake the role they want me to do, or they worry that trying to do so much will affect my mental health and cause me to burn out.

On the other hand, other employers have felt that my various roles, work experience (including the projects I have initiated) makes me innovative and useful in providing feedback and suggesting new ways of working for their organisation.

Despite what some potential employers might think, I believe that the majority of my experiences bring something to the roles I am applying for. My experiences demonstrate my journey and everything I have learnt along the way; I am immensely proud of them and the career they have allowed me to develop. I believe that most enlightened employers have a positive view of a varied CV such as mine!

Remember that you can and should always tailor your CV and covering letter to the role you are applying for. I generally keep my CV the same most of the time though, and just highlight relevant areas in my covering letter (of course you must also explain any gaps on your CV).

multiple places (even if in industry-related areas) might be viewed negatively by some employers because it may make you look fickle or unsure about what you want out of your career. The chances of this in a linear medical career are of course slim because we usually follow a straightforward training pathway. However, in some cases trainees might have had several years out of training (gap years are becoming more commonplace now, though) or may have changed specialties once or twice. A GP might move around several practices before they find somewhere they want to settle in the long term. Being able to justify your decisions and explain your thought processes is one way to potentially overcome this issue. You could do this by briefly detailing your reasons for leaving somewhere on the application form, or at the interview or another occasion where you have the chance to speak to a prospective employer or colleague, perhaps on an informal basis.

Gain relevant work experience (even if this might be difficult to do!)

Gain work experience in the areas of interest to you and in areas that will impact your future job prospects (both directly and indirectly, for example, via transferable skills).

The obvious way to do this is by applying for work in relevant roles, even if you do not meet all the essential criteria. However, your chances may be slim if employers do not feel you have sufficient human capital to completely fulfil the requirements of the role. Of course, you could always seek out opportunities to shadow others and speak to colleagues to gain additional insight and experience. Let's use an example to illustrate this point.

Perhaps you want to join a GP partnership. GP practices may place more weighting on an experienced GP, because as a newly qualified GP you probably know little about running a business, and so you may not feel confident applying for such roles. However, if you do apply, the practice might consider you a suitable candidate because of your experience, achievements and transferable skills (such as leadership) in other clinical and non-clinical roles, even if these may not include running a business. So, it is still worth applying. If you do not feel ready to apply for such roles then you may struggle to make significant progress with your career.

When I applied for a future partnership role, I was seen to have potential and lots of relevant clinical and non-clinical experience. I was offered a partnership within two years (the length of time was a combination of needing further experience, getting to know the staff and financial factors). So, despite not having specific experience in running a GP surgery, my varied experience was seen as beneficial and helped me secure the role.

Can you list three ways to gain meaningful work experience in areas of interest to you?

Example – I can list three companies in aesthetic medicine where I can apply for jobs / email my CV / arrange a meeting to shadow some of the doctors, which might lead to a job (somewhere!)

Section summary

- Human capital is a broad term; it encompasses a variety of areas that will improve your value when applying for jobs or seeking out new opportunities.
- Your medical education, additional postgraduate qualifications and a suitable amount of work experience are all important factors in ensuring you can create a career that will provide you with your version of success.
- Employers (or clients and customers) place a significant weighting on your qualifications and work experience – so think about how you can outshine your competitors. How can you become more competent and experienced and then demonstrate this?

3.4 Self-help tools for successful career planning and development

Whichever way you choose to define career success, you'll need to do some career planning. There are multiple ways to do this; if you don't feel that you can manage this planning by yourself, then there are many sources of help available, such as coaching, counselling, or self-help guides on the internet. I thought it would be appropriate to provide you with some 'self-help' aids outlined in an article by Robert C. Reardon. These prompts can be used on their own or with additional support, such as courses or careers counselling; you might decide to use a combination depending on how self-directed you are (whether you need lots of help or not).

I have set out below the two key elements for you to consider as you get started with planning your career:

- **Career planning readiness:** are you ready to start career planning?
- **Awareness of the options:** do you clearly know what options are available and right for you?

3.4.1 Career planning readiness

Making a decision (likely a big one) about your career requires you to be **ready**, which will allow you to make the best use of what is around you (i.e. resources and people) and so increase your chances of success in creating the right career for you.

Cast your mind back to *Section 2.2*, where we initially discussed that the first step in creating a portfolio career is career planning readiness. The literature surrounding career planning looks at whether an individual is *ready* to participate in this process and, if they are, *how* they go about doing this. If an individual is unsure about who they are and what they would like to do, then they may need the additional help of someone like a careers counsellor. However, if an individual has clarity about who they are and what they would like to do, then they may be more suited to using self-help resources. By working through this book, you may have already begun to develop an idea of what your portfolio career would look like, so self-help resources may well be sufficient for you. The benefits of self-help include working through resources in your own time, around other commitments, and reducing the cost of any private counselling or courses. I had a few sessions through

Health Education England (HEE) during my time out of training after the foundation programme. These sessions were useful, especially when used in conjunction with self-help resources and lived experiences, i.e. making decisions and learning from those and so pivoting away from or towards a particular area.

Assessing your career planning readiness

- What do you think your level of readiness is?

- Have you asked yourself if you are **truly** ready to make decisions regarding your career?

Some factors, such as the ones set out below, may be affecting your level of readiness and thus your ability to use resources adequately.

Personal characteristics: *such as negative thoughts and feelings which can be acute and/or chronic.* Are you someone who struggles to see the positive side of things? Do you have a background of depression or anxiety? If so, perhaps a good starting point would be trying to address negative thoughts before developing your career.

Personal circumstances: *your lived experiences.* What is going on in your life right now? Have you had a bereavement? Have you recently changed jobs? Are you having problems at home? What are your finances like? Do you foresee a time when you might be more able to dedicate a significant proportion of time to career planning?

Awareness level: *an awareness about yourself and the options and resources available that can help with making career decisions.*

Are you confident you know yourself well? Do you know what opportunities exist and which ones might be open to you? Have you got a plan, in your head or on paper, that lists the opportunities available and where you will go to get help to target those opportunities?

Figure 3.1 is the first self-help aid to help you decide on the level of support you need based on your career readiness level.

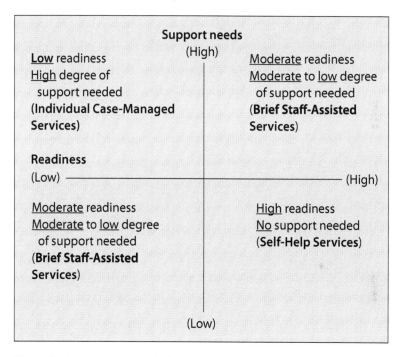

Figure 3.1 *Assessing your level of career planning readiness and the support you need.*

3.4.2 Awareness of the options

When making a choice about your career, the cognitive information processing pyramid (*Figure 3.2*) can be used so you know **where** to focus. You may feel that you know yourself quite well, especially after having completed the exercises in *Chapter 2*. However, you may not be aware of the various options open to you, or how you make vital decisions. *Where do you need to focus your attention first?*

Use this second aid to home in on what is missing in your pyramid.

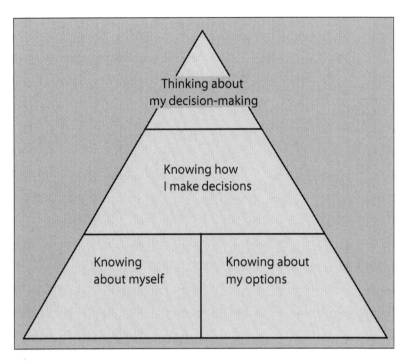

Figure 3.2 What to consider when making career decisions.

The Self-Directed Search (SDS) Interpretive Report details six personality types and indicates various occupations and areas of study based on these groupings (see the RIASEC hexagon in *Figure 3.3*). Individuals who spent more time reading through the report spent more time considering possible options and considering a wider range of occupations. But once those individuals fully understood themselves in relation to the working environment, they were able to narrow down their possible choices to a more limited range of occupations.

Take a moment to review the RIASEC hexagon:

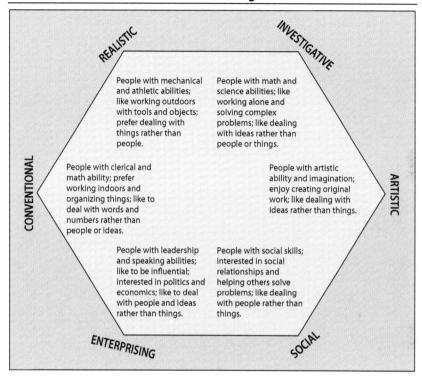

Figure 3.3 *RIASEC hexagon.*

- Where do you fit into the hexagon?

- Do you resonate with more than one characteristic / occupation?

- How does this correspond to your stable individual characteristics (the 'Big Five' introduced to you in *Section 3.2.3*)?

Understanding yourself (your skills, qualities, abilities, strengths, weaknesses, personality type) is key to creating your portfolio career!

- Start by researching a broad range of options (jobs and pathways) and then narrowing them down based on **what you know about yourself** and what could **be possible** for you:
  - how much time in the past have you spent considering possible options?
  - do you need to dedicate more or less time?

- You will spend less time deciding **what to do** if you have a clear focus on the **specific areas** of interest **suited to you and your unique circumstances**.
  - how could you go about searching for more information in your areas of interest?

Section summary

- Creating a portfolio career requires proper planning. Whilst this may not be a rigid plan of exactly what you want to do, you should have a clear idea of what you'd like your career to look like.
- Before you jump into creating a sound plan, you need to consider if you are ready to begin this process. Career readiness involves you reviewing your personal characteristics, your unique circumstances, and your awareness level.
- Your level of career planning readiness will determine whether you need one-to-one help or if self-help resources are sufficient.
- Self-help aids include the CIP pyramid and RIASEC hexagon. The CIP pyramid helps you know where you need to focus, whilst the RIASEC hexagon helps you match your personality to a working environment.
- Self-help aids may be more suited to those who feel fairly confident they know themselves well. They can be used in conjunction with other methods such as careers coaching, or on their own.

3.5 Identifying what additional support and (social) skills you need to stand out

The final component within human capital is social capital. Given that there is a significant amount of information in this section, I have summarised the main learning points, such that you will be able to:

- recognise that social capital is a complex construct with several important aspects that cannot be ignored for a successful portfolio career
- understand social network compositions and how these can be created, developed and effectively utilised in portfolio career creation
- analyse your own social networks by thinking about how you can maximise the existing relationships you have and foster newer ones.

3.5.1 What is social capital?

There is no single definition for social capital. It is commonly viewed as social organisations, networks or groups (which may differ in size and importance) that exist to bring about positive changes for both individuals and society. Of course, theories relating to social capital have their flaws; for example, there may not always be positive effects on those outside of the group. Remember, the focus is how you can apply these ideas to your own career. So, let's look at social networks and *why* these are important.

3.5.2 The structure of social networks

Theories pertaining to *social networks* look at the relationships or 'ties' between individuals in a combination of ties also known as a network. We all exist within numerous and often diverse social networks. The networks or ties between our friends, for example, are stronger than those between our acquaintances – called 'weak ties' (hence *'weak tie theory'* outlined by Granovetter in 1973). Weak ties can function as connections or entry points to other networks (including individuals from diverse backgrounds) and provide different types of information not found within a network of strong ties. A good example of this would be the potential access to financial advice from a different social network.

Another term, 'structural holes' describes how the central person in a network (yourself or 'ego'; see *Figure 3.4*) should have several connections or ties ('alters') who are not connected or related to each other. This helps the person at the centre of this network in several ways:

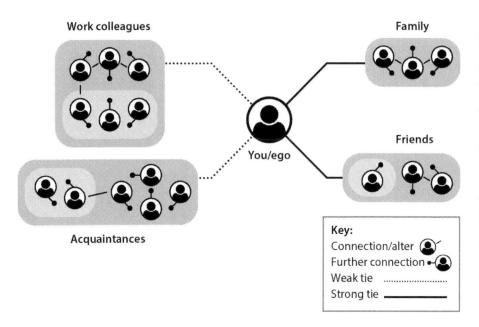

Figure 3.4 A visual representation of the different social networks someone may be a part of, showing alters and ego. Usually those in our networks will know and/or be related to one another.

- Information sharing
  - they can acquire various types of information and potentially access it more rapidly
  - they might have greater 'control' over the information because of exclusivity (access to information others may not have access to)

- The ability to negotiate because of their advantage within the networks
  - this might lead to a greater influence over resources

- Greater visibility
- More opportunities for their career.

Thus, it seems to make sense to have more structural holes in your network. Recognising where those structural holes are, who you have strong and weak ties with, enables you to accurately focus your time and energy.

Finally, *social resources theory* looks specifically at the *resources* within a network. This includes the resources a connection can provide, such as access to additional and varied information, financial support and credibility. For example, if you would like more information regarding a particular occupation, then you might reach out to a contact who is in that field or potentially knows someone else who is. Interestingly, according to this theory, weak ties are associated with those who are society's elites, and having lots of weak ties could therefore improve the calibre of job you could secure.

To summarise, social networks (with various structures as above) can provide the following benefits for those involved:

- A supply of plentiful resources which includes new, exclusive, varied and significant amounts of information; that access to information could be rapid, which might help with changing careers or creating innovative ideas and projects

- Career success, through access to contacts in more senior positions within an organisation and from *different* organisations; this includes career sponsorship or mentoring (discussed in more detail in *Section 3.6*)

- An additional benefit includes simply engaging with others for human interaction! This may also involve trying to maintain existing relationships with contacts from previous events or with work colleagues.

Taking the time to understand the networks you are in and how you can nurture them is a crucial part of ensuring you have (and can give back) what is needed to create a successful portfolio career.

Here are a few questions to consider regarding social networks:

- How **many** social networks do you have?
  - think about personal, professional, extracurricular, online and offline

- What **types** of individuals are in your networks, and do you have weak or strong ties to them?
  - think about their personality type, occupation and any personal details they may have shared with you, e.g. whether they have siblings, a partner, etc.
  - who do you have strong ties with?
  - who do you have weak ties with?

- Why do you **value** your network(s)?

- Do you think your social network contains the **connections** and **resources** you need to reach the level of career success you desire?

- What could you do to **improve** your networks? How could you develop or nurture personal or professional relationships? Could you provide something beneficial too? Could you reciprocate, i.e. provide information relevant to someone else's career if they have done so for yours? Could you invite someone out for a meal if they have previously bought you lunch?

- Importantly, which relationships are important for you to **invest** your time and effort into? Do you want to invest significant amounts of energy into creating a small number of really strong ties or many weak ties, or a combination of both? It might be worth deciding which ones you want to focus on. Perhaps initially creating several weak ties (through attending events in a field you are interested in) and then homing in on those you want to strengthen. I will discuss more about how you can do this through my networking tips and advice in *Section 3.5.3*.

- Would you consider any of those in your networks as **mentors**? If so, why? If not, what can you do to change this? Research has shown that those with multiple mentors have greater levels of career success.

You can use the template in *Figure 3.5* to help you think about the questions above, and start to identify gaps, such as missing connections or resources you still need access to.

3.5.3 What networking is and how to do it well

This next section will cover:

- how you can enhance your social networks – by improving existing ones and cultivating new relationships with others
- how to successfully network with others.

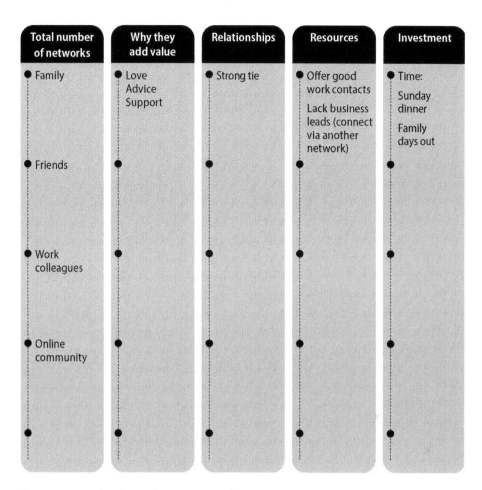

Total number of networks	Why they add value	Relationships	Resources	Investment
● Family	● Love Advice Support	● Strong tie	● Offer good work contacts Lack business leads (connect via another network)	● Time: Sunday dinner Family days out
● Friends	●	●	●	●
● Work colleagues	●	●	●	●
● Online community	●	●	●	●
●	●	●	●	●

Figure 3.5 *Template for analysing your social networks.*

Ways to improve your social networks

So, we have covered some of the reasons *why* social networks (and networking) are important. Building on this, social networks can be a great way to listen to and learn from other people's stories. By speaking to others, it might also help you understand what gaps there could be, i.e. what the needs of a certain group are and how you might be able to address those needs through your own portfolio. You could also use the contacts within the various networks to test out new ideas or hypotheses about what might or might not work in your career. Some of the contacts in your network could also become business partners or team members. An important point to mention here is that networking or being a part of social networks should be about exchanging information and resources for mutual benefit. I will discuss the ways you can do this shortly.

Now, let's look at *how* you can improve your social networks and networking skills.

Networking will help you build your social networks in terms of size, quality, strength of connections and resources

Networking is the process of building a meaningful connection with someone, whether that is a long- or short-term connection (or a strong or weak tie) that can benefit you both in some way.

If you think about the strongest ties in your social networks – your parents, siblings, your best friends – you will realise that you have deep connections with them that developed over several years. The likelihood is that you would help them if they needed something and they would most likely do the same for you (within reason of course!). Although you may not be able to make such strong connections with other people whom you might meet during an evening, you can gradually begin to formulate professional relationships with others over time.

Connections

What makes you stay connected with some people and not others?

What makes you want to share information that could benefit others in your network?

When you meet someone for the first time, someone that you would like to learn more about because, for example, their career is inspiring or they have an interesting array of roles, think about what you can do to leave a lasting impression. *How can you reconnect with them to see if there is the potential to build a strong professional relationship or tie in your network?* Not everyone will become strong ties, but being able to keep them in your network as perhaps a weak tie and focusing on others who might become strong ties is one way to continue to build your network.

I have provided you with some idea of what I believe networking to be. As you can see, it is a fairly broad term, but I hope you will understand why it needs to be when reading the next point. However, because it is such a broad term you will need to be much more specific when it comes to detailing what you want to achieve when participating in different social networks and networking opportunities.

When, where and with whom should I network?

There are always opportunities to network, they are everywhere. You just need to identify and make the most out of them.

- *When: all the time; at every opportunity!*

Whether we realise it or not, we are networking and building social networks most of the time: with our close friends and families or when we are at work or go to social events. I used opportunities during teaching sessions as a trainee to network with the speakers. This may have involved asking more about their company or their specialist interest. Other examples in more immediate networks could be a friend who introduced you to someone and now you and that person are extremely close. That person is now in one of your social networks. The conversations you have with family and friends, perhaps those discussing a new venture, could develop because someone in your network might know someone who could help you. So, be on the lookout for opportunities wherever you go.

Often when the word networking is used, one might think of going to several events and building lots of contacts quickly. Although this is one way to network, it is not the only way; it can be very time-consuming and if there is a lack of clear goals or reasons for networking it can be a truly pointless exercise. Networking on a smaller, more individual and personal scale may reap better and longer-lasting results, depending on your personality type, your interest and the goals you have. However, if you network predominantly by attending events, make sure you have a clear strategy for how you will make the most of the events and choose the right ones based on your interests, the skills you want to develop and the fields you want to break into. I go into more detail below about what you can do at events to maximise their benefits.

You should also think about how to optimise your time and energy. Networking after a long day at work might be too tiring. Perhaps selecting one evening or a day off every month for attending events could be an idea?

Recurring events or joining groups that meet up regularly could also help.

- *Where: everywhere! There are always opportunities to network. For more focused networking, you can try contacting individuals within and outside of your network via social media, websites, email and phone, attending events and joining groups online and offline.*

Based on the information you have hopefully compiled during the previous chapters, you should have some idea of your fields of interest and what you would like to add to (or remove from) your portfolio career. For example, if you are interested in digital health, you may want to make a list of the *places* (both online and offline) that you should be visiting to network and increase your contacts in this area. You might want to start with a broad search in your local area and define a certain area you are willing (and have the time and money) to travel within. You might want to then whittle it down based on what is specific to your needs. Sites such as Eventbrite and Meetup can be helpful as well as LinkedIn and Facebook. It might seem time-consuming, and indeed it can be initially, but if you have a clear focus, it should hopefully make things easier as time goes on.

There are many events online and, whilst I would encourage a combination of both offline and online events, I personally think in-person events are much better ways to build a rapport and increase your chances of building more meaningful connections.

- *Who: existing contacts and networks (those outside of your social networks too) – in your areas of interest, working in the roles you see yourself in. Also individuals working in areas you may not have considered previously and in unrelated fields.*

> I want you to realise that there are lots of opportunities to add to your existing networks and strengthen 'weak ties'.

Before looking at building connections with 'new' people, it might be worth considering people you already know. You can start by looking through the contacts in your phone, addresses in your email inbox, and/or looking at the places you have worked or volunteered at, to see if there is anyone you know who you may want to contact again. You might yield some surprising results. This is one way to potentially strengthen 'weak ties'. Don't forget your family and friends! We can gain lots of different types of support from our existing networks such as practical (looking after the kids for a few hours), financial (helping us with completing our tax returns), emotional (a shoulder to lean on after a hard day), etc.

You should also make a list of the *people* you want to contact, whether by attending their events, or making direct contact with them (if you feel confident to do so) and arranging a meeting online and/or in person. You can contact them via their social media profiles or they may have a website where you can complete a 'contact form' or send them an email. When making a list, consider what their roles or job titles are and learn more about what this means, i.e. what they do day-to-day in their role. As above, you may be able to attend their events, invite them to yours or potentially shadow them in their role(s).

It is also important to think about contacting those in unrelated fields. Be open-minded when networking. A trap I see many medics fall into (including myself at times…) is staying within medical social networks. Whilst this is common, it might hinder your progress. For example, if you want to start a business the medics in your network may have no idea about how to do this. You may have to consider broadening your network to include those who can help you in this area.

My '4 Ps' to excellent networking

Networking is a skill that can be learnt. You may not know exactly where to start, or you may have an idea and experience but want to further enhance and refine your skills. By following the steps shown in *Figure 3.6*, which are a combination of my own personal experiences and research, you will have a good formula for networking success.

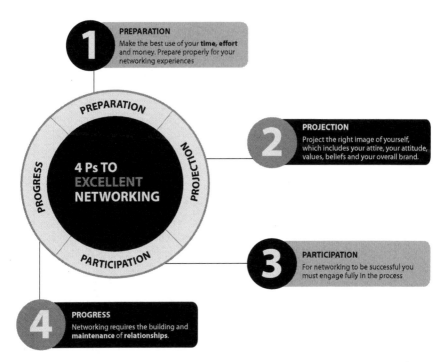

Figure 3.6 *The '4 Ps' to excellent networking – a process which requires consistent effort, collaboration and trust.*

1. Preparation

Like most things in life, I believe preparation is key. Taking a little bit more time to plan your steps can make a massive impact on your overall results.

Before you read on, spend a few moments writing down why you personally want (or need) to network.

Why network?

I want to network because *(here's an example to get you started)*:

1. It will allow me to access new information

2.

3.

One of your main aims is to ensure you use your time wisely and meet the right contacts who will help you develop your portfolio career. So, before going to lots of events (because they seem interesting or you have been advised to by friends) do your research. This will help you develop the *quality* of social networks needed to progress your career.

You might find it helpful to divide the places you can network into the following:

- Your organisation
  - For example, if you work in a GP surgery you might want to ask if there are any new audits of Quality Improvement Projects (QIPs) you can assist someone with. You could ask about starting your own and ask colleagues to help. You could also attend social events or buy a thank you card for a colleague who has helped you.

- Your profession
  - Attending learning events advertised by the BMA, the *British Medical Journal* (BMJ) or the Royal College of General Practitioners, or undertaking a voluntary role at the BMA or part-time role on the Integrated Care Board (ICB).

- Other specialties and professions
  - Offer your expertise via speaking engagements or through articles. You could also attend events at other Royal Colleges such as the Royal College of Obstetricians and Gynaecologists or even completely outside of the medical field.

- Your community
  - You could serve as a school governor, volunteer at or become a trustee of a charity.

Now, let's look at how you can prepare for a standard conference. It will have a theme, speakers, and stands and stalls for exhibitors. In the run-up to the event there will usually be several emails detailing the programme, including information about the speakers and their topics, the advertisers, exhibitors and more. You will therefore have ample time to prepare; think about what you want to gain from the event and how you can achieve this. You don't want to miss out on potential opportunities! At the same time, remember that it should be fun so be cautious about being too meticulous and rigid in your planning.

Things to think about:

- Which speakers will you be interested in listening to? Which ones not so much?

- If you decide to miss a talk, is there an opportunity to visit the stands and speak to exhibitors or others also attending the event instead?

- How can you engage with technology before the event (if available) such as apps or forums to learn more about attendees?

2. Projection

- Your personality:

As we saw in *Section 3.2.3*, there are different personality types. Some individuals are more open to meeting new people and/or looking for new experiences than others (extroversion and openness to experience, respectively). So, for those who are this way inclined, networking may come more naturally. If this is not you, don't worry because you can learn how to network effectively. Understanding which personality types have been linked to career success will help you understand more about yourself and how you can improve your level of career success, i.e. through your approach to networking.

Many of us probably fit on a spectrum and exhibit some characteristics of all (or most) of the Big Five personality types ('neuroticism', 'conscientiousness', 'extroversion', 'agreeableness' and 'openness to experience').

For instance, someone who is conscientious might be very proactive, thriving even if their environment is challenging. They go above and beyond at work, use their initiative and are determined to bring about change in a meaningful way.

Proactive individuals do not wait for change; they initiate it.

Think about how you can be more proactive when it comes to networking, your career and even your personal life.

- Your attitude

The ABC (Affect, Cognition, Behaviour) model of ambivalence is useful when reflecting on your attitude, especially towards networking.

Many of our associations with objects or people (colleagues, partners / spouses) are a combination of both positive and negative thoughts, beliefs and feelings. This is called 'attitudinal ambivalence' (*importantly, the negative aspects of an ambivalent attitude have more weighting*).

According to the ABC model, and Theory of Planned Behaviour (TPB), there are three factors or consequences to an ambivalent attitude:

- **cognitive** – what we believe
- **affective** – how we feel
- **behavioural** – how we act.

So, your attitude towards networking and the people you encounter during networking activities is a combination of these factors, and this has implications on what you believe, how you feel and how you act.

You may have had negative experiences with networking in the past and so have a mixture of emotions and thoughts about it as a result. This may then influence your choices about attending future events; you may decline opportunities that could be valuable for you and your career. You should try to understand *why* your experience was not a positive one and then consider *what you can do* at a future event to turn it into a more positive experience.

Make a list of any negatives and turn them into positives (*I've added an example to get you started*):

Negative experience and why	How can this be a positive one?
"I did not meet any potential contacts" • Perhaps I did not make a conscious effort to smile and appear approachable or I did not initiate conversation.	I can appear approachable by smiling and using more eye contact. I can say hello to someone and ask them what they thought about the talk. If I think we have a few things in common and could continue the conversation I will ask them for a means to contact them, e.g. their email address or LinkedIn profile.

By reading on hopefully you will be able to reflect more on the *why* and implement some of the tips below to make future networking eventful!

• Your professional demeanour:

As doctors we should all be familiar with the GMC's *Good Medical Practice* which details how we should act as a medical professional. The GMC has also provided guidance regarding professionalism beyond clinical practice, such as when using social media.

Professionalism can be linked to a set of values and behaviours, and understanding these behaviours helps if you are looking for feedback on performance (because it is more objective). Start by reviewing the examples of values and behaviours below. Put them into practice daily, which of course includes during your time at an event (you may want to review your value and beliefs in *Section 2.4.4*). This is a key step in making a great first impression.

- *Responsibility* – you can demonstrate this by being on time for the event and any specific activities that occur during the event, such as speed networking, talks or group tasks. It also helps in any networking activities you engage with (to build trust and develop collaborative working) by completing tasks as agreed and holding yourself accountable for any mistakes you have made.
- *Communication skills and maturity* – you should actively listen to the person you are trying to connect with; open body language and good eye contact show the other person you are listening. Also be patient, which you can demonstrate by not interrupting the other person when they speak.
- *Respect* – show respect to everyone you interact with, regardless of their level or role within an organisation.

• Personal branding:

Personal branding is still a relatively new concept which has its origins in marketing. The need to understand and develop a personal brand has developed alongside the rise in social media platforms and the increase in remote working. Personal branding requires you to make a *conscious effort* to work *strategically* on creating a *positive image* of yourself for career success. This positive image needs to convey a *unique message* of *how* you can *help* those you are marketing yourself to, i.e. your *target audience*.

Personal branding should be thought of as a critical career tool or proactive work behaviour that can help improve your level of career success. Here are some questions to ask yourself which will help with creating and conveying your personal brand:

• Your *professional image* and how you analyse it:
- How do you demonstrate your professional image in person and online? *For example, showcasing your employment history (via social media or professional websites) through a fully completed profile. Perhaps you can lead community events or organise a fundraising initiative. This is a good way to support*

charitable causes, simultaneously gain lots of skills and present yourself in a positive light.
- Do you regularly present your professional image to your network and then evaluate how you do this? *For example, do you post consistently on LinkedIn and review the analytics regarding engagement?*
- Are you selective in the type of information you share with those within and outside of your networks? *For example, you could consider sharing things that have gone less well for you, as well as your successes.*

• Your *professional activity* including what sets you apart from others (your unique selling point or USP):
  - Do you regularly attend networking events within and outside of your profession and/or organisation? *For example, how many work socials or health conferences have you attended in the past year?*

> You can always offer something when networking, i.e. you may not be an 'expert' but you can certainly make a contribution. You have more resources than you know! For example, you might know someone in your network that could be of assistance to your new contact, or you could offer a positive outlook and encouragement.

  - Do you try to differentiate yourself from others? *For example, do you list your areas of interest, specialties or achievements on your own professional website? Do you provide specific evidence of your work and how you are different? What is your area of expertise? Is your area of expertise or the way in which you can help others clear in all your communication? Here's an example of clear communication:* "I offer bespoke careers coaching services to professionals who want to improve their knowledge and ability to prevent burnout. Roughly x% of traditional coaching services **do not focus** specifically on preventing burnout. **This is where I'm different.**" *(Find a statistic relating to your own area of expertise and use this, to illustrate how you or your service are different).*
  - Do you ask for professional recommendations and endorsements from those in your networks? *For example, do you obtain feedback from work colleagues? Do you ask for recommendations on LinkedIn? Do you ask others to endorse the list of skills on your LinkedIn profile? It is much better to have your contacts speak positively about you and recommend you rather than you doing this yourself (all the time).*

Conveying your personal brand involves some level of social media usage and if you are not familiar with social media or have hesitations about using it, I suggest you rethink. You really should use social media, but use it carefully and consult the GMC's guidance in the first instance.

There are several social media platforms you can use for professional purposes, but LinkedIn should be viewed as one of the best ways to convey your personal brand, network and look for job opportunities (both freelance and employed work). There are many benefits associated with using LinkedIn, so let's briefly discuss what these are and how you can start thinking about using it more effectively.

At the time of writing there are, according to LinkedIn, roughly 850 million members across every country in the world using the platform. This provides a huge database of users who you can search for (and who can search for you!) and connect with based on your aims and interests. If a LinkedIn profile is completed fully and accurately and updated regularly, you can learn lots about someone (and they can learn lots about you too); for example, the services they provide, the skills they have acquired and their accomplishments. This can help you quickly gather significant amounts of information depending on what you need or who you want to connect with. You can also learn who and which organisations they are connected with, including who they work for. Other useful features include joining groups and searching for jobs.

Networking via LinkedIn can lead to gaining more contacts, but remember that more contacts does not always equal active, engaged members of your network. Furthermore, *regular use* can provide access to new information, ideas and career sponsorship. Interestingly, however, there does not seem to be much benefit in using LinkedIn for social support, which is better gained from in-person interactions.

> If you want to develop a portfolio career, then you need to be proactive; seek out new opportunities, create your own and challenge your current circumstances!

We know that social media can have both positive and negative effects on both our professional and personal lives. Whilst I am not going to list all the risks associated with using the internet, including social media, I think it is useful to share a few key tips for using social media wisely because these points may not be obvious to everyone (see *Appendix 2: Social media tips*).

3. Participation (interaction)

To make the most out of networking you need to fully engage in the process, especially if you are not able to attend many events. Use the list of suggestions below to help you make the most of the networking activity you attend:

- **Create a strong first impression** – make eye contact and smile, and try to ensure you have a good firm handshake and speak clearly; if you don't (or can't) shake someone's hand, then the other three tips are even more important!
- **Initiate conversation** – don't be afraid of rejection! Start with open-ended questions just like you would when talking to a patient; here are a few suggestions you might want to use if you get stuck:
  - *"What was your main reason for attending today?"*
  - *"What are you looking forward to doing/who are you looking forward to hearing from the most today?"*
  - *"Have you attended an event like this/one of these events before?"*

It can be difficult to break into an already formed group of people, so try to be punctual and start conversations before larger groups have formed.

> Build a rapport – remember that networking is a two-way process and so think about genuinely building a connection with someone rather than simply working out what you can use them for.

- **Be clear, specific and concise about who you are, what you can offer and what you need help with** – this may also be known as the 'elevator pitch' or '30 second commercial'.
  - *Who are you? What is your professional background, skills and experience in a nutshell?*
  - *What do you offer and why is it different? (i.e. what is your USP? What makes you stand out from the crowd?)*
  - *What are you looking for? Do you need financial support or help with navigating the business world or both? Are you looking for a co-founder, investor, a team or all of the above?*
- **Stay engaged, enthusiastic and curious** – actively listen to what the person has to say. Try repeating what you have heard (and

using their name in conversation) to demonstrate you are truly listening – this helps build rapport; find some commonalities in addition to working out how you can add value to their network when following up (see below). Try to keep the conversation going by asking lots of open questions and don't focus too much on yourself!

- **Keep it moving** – don't fall into the trap of staying with one or two people or a group for the duration of the event. Similarly, if you do attend with someone you know, you might want to split up for at least a portion of the event. If you want to move on to speak to someone else, you could try connecting people together or simply politely excuse yourself.

4. Progress (follow-up)

The main aim of networking is to build long-term professional relationships (through reconnecting), so try to build stronger ties with those you seemed to connect with at the event. Studies have found that the follow-up rate after an event ranges from 20 to 42%. This may demonstrate: (1) a lack of value provided by the event organisers; (2) that participants did not make enough 'valuable' connections (or struggled to network at online events); or (3) that participants did not grasp how a potential contact could become a strong tie or long-term connection. If follow-up rates after events are generally quite poor, perhaps attendees struggle with *how* to effectively reconnect with others after an event? Follow-up rates might be improved if organisers could create specific events to reconnect, share email addresses (with consent) and encourage the use of platforms such as Slack, WhatsApp or LinkedIn. *But none of this should stop you from following up!*

Learning about your contacts will ultimately help you to decide whether you share common values, beliefs and interests. Working collaboratively on projects and helping one another will help build trust over time, therefore strengthening ties and forming strong professional relationships. So, here are a few tips:

- Make a list (soon after the event) of who you encountered and key points about them, including what they said – this is good so in subsequent encounters you can show them that you listened and remembered things about them and their business / work.
- Think about how you could mutually benefit each other, or whether there are any opportunities to work together.

- Follow up with an email / text message / phone or video call depending on level of appropriateness. You can also use social media platforms such as LinkedIn and X (previously Twitter) which may have been used to help engagement prior to and during the event. Contacting individuals via virtual methods can be useful initially, especially if you are more of an introverted person.
- Secure a follow-up meeting and, if all goes well, ensure you continue to offer value by:
  - sending them relevant information such as websites, articles, courses, events, and contacts who might be useful.
  - letting them know how you might be able to help them – how your expertise can help them with their problem (if they have one). They might also remember you when speaking to someone else and create referrals for your services.

So, those are the '4 Ps' to excellent networking. You should re-read them until you feel you can confidently network in different settings. A top tip would be to re-read them just before an event and pick one or two areas to focus on during the event.

Section summary

- You are in numerous social networks which include family, friends, work colleagues and acquaintances.
- Learn how to harness the power of social networks – creating more 'structural holes' may help you gain access to lots more information and resources than you would have had access to otherwise.
- Consistently engage with others; think about cultivating new relationships outside of your familiar networks.
- Don't be afraid to network with new people – use my '4 Ps' to help you do this successfully.
- Be careful about how you use various methods to network, such as social media.

3.6 How your organisation can help you

3.6.1 What is mentoring and sponsorship?

The final key predictor to discuss is organisational sponsorship. So, let's now look at how the organisation(s) you are part of can support your career development. In this section I will also cover mentoring, where a mentor is an experienced individual who can support and advise you over a long period of time.

Cast your mind back to *Section 3.2.2*, when we first looked at contest and sponsored mobility. Your career success is not just your ability to work hard but also the level of support you receive in the form of sponsorship. Think of organisational sponsorship as an umbrella term encompassing support from individuals and resources available through your organisation.

The terms 'mentoring' and 'sponsoring' are often used interchangeably but, as you will see, sponsorship goes that one step further than mentoring. Sponsorship helps to ensure you reach your level of success instead of simply steering you in the direction you think you should go.

Understanding the difference

Be aware of the various terms used regarding mentoring, and where they sit on the spectrum:

- 'Developmental mentoring' – the mentor takes on a more supportive role, guiding the mentee on their own path. This is the least assertive form of mentoring.
- 'Sponsorship mentoring', as described above – the mentor takes more of the lead in the mentoring relationship; actively promoting the mentee and providing opportunities for them. This is a somewhat assertive form of mentoring.
- 'Talent management mentoring' – the mentor takes even more control than in 'sponsorship mentoring', creating a plan for the mentee, advocating for them and providing significant levels of support within the organisation. This is the most assertive form of mentoring.

Factors affecting organisational sponsorship include whether:

- support is available from senior colleagues, mentors and supervisors
- opportunities exist to participate in training exercises and activities to develop new and existing skills
- the organisation has sufficient resources available (this is usually related to its size).

You should think about these factors in relation to where you work or where you would like to work in the future. Let's look at a GP surgery, for example:

- Do the senior staff have a track record of supporting their employees?
  - *do they book staff bonding days or team exercises?*
  - *do they arrange social events like lunch or evening meals occasionally?*
  - *have they supported staff emotionally if needed?*
- Is the practice supportive when it comes to developing its employees' skills?
  - *is there provision for educational grants or time for study leave?*
  - *is there time for clinical discussions or case-based meetings?*
- How big is the practice?
  - *a bigger practice might have the space and budget for practical procedures and interventions, and so more training.*

In addition to thinking carefully about how your organisation can support you in the ways above, you may want to start thinking about how you can contribute to your organisation. This could result in you standing out from the crowd and being *selected* for sponsorship within your organisation (i.e. a suitable mentor might want to support you). Here are two suggestions that can help you get 'selected':

- Creating the right image:
  - diligence: you may want to put yourself forward for challenging tasks
  - teamwork: you could offer support to fellow colleagues; for example, completing additional work if a staff member is ill
  - willing to learn and listen to advice: be ready to take on board constructive feedback and be open to suggestions
  - innovation: what about suggesting ideas for improvements at the practice, such as a patient focus group or ways to implement patient feedback?
- Working on your personality type: recognise those aspects of your individual differences or personality that might be hindering your level of success, and see what you can do to change them. I know I am not the most positive of people so over the years I have worked hard to change my outlook – I work hard at it most days, but I am much better now!

3.6.2 How can you find and approach a potential mentor?

Before we take a deep dive into how you get started with approaching a mentor, it is important to highlight here some pertinent points:

- *Don't get too bogged down with finding that one 'right' person –* I do not believe that there is one person who can adequately support you in all areas of a mentoring relationship. Therefore, rather than focusing on one particular person, look for the skills, qualities and experience in more than one mentor. Perhaps you will need to speak to one mentor when you feel you need careers coaching and another when you are looking for more emotional support.

- Following on from the above, *do not be restricted in where you are looking for a mentor.* For example, you may look for a mentoring relationship with the GP partner you are working for; they can support you with your clinical work and understanding how a GP surgery is run as a business. However, you may want to look outside of a clinical setting for a mentor who can help you with the non-clinical aspects or roles in your portfolio career; for example, a mentor with expertise in marketing or personal branding.

Example 3.3 – You don't need the 'right' person, you need multiple mentors

I am currently part of the NHS Clinical Entrepreneur Programme (CEP) which enables me to receive a structured approach to mentoring, and I also gained a mentor as part of the Emerging Women Leaders Programme (see *Example 2.1*). I have been a part of both formal and informal mentoring, which was based on me actively looking for a mentor. Instead of trying to find the 'right' mentor (which is how I used to look at it), think about what you can learn from each person you encounter. You might find, like myself, that being a part of a formal programme is much better or even complements the informal mentoring you might receive from colleagues.

Evidence shows that having a mentor or mentors is beneficial to your career and also to the organisation. The mentor might offer you support with starting a new job, networking, achieving your goals, professionalism, personal development and research. Another way to look at the benefits of mentoring would be via the talent management mentoring wheel (by Merrick and Stokes, 2008; see *Figure 3.7*) which provides a good summary:

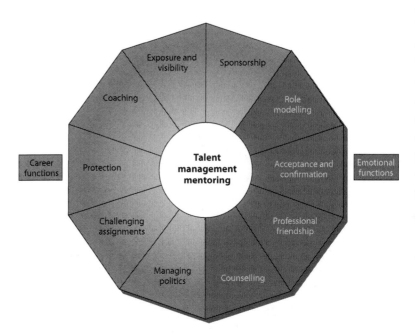

Figure 3.7 *The talent management mentoring wheel, summarising the benefits of this type of mentoring relationship.*

There should also be benefits for the mentor, such as fulfilment, accomplishment, development of leadership skills and recognition at work in the form of promotions and awards; you may want to bear this in mind when approaching a potential mentor (see also the additional tips below).

Before you approach a potential mentor think carefully about why you are looking for one.

Think about specific reasons for wanting a mentor (*I've added a couple of examples to get you started*):

How to build connections in the pharmaceutical industry

Developing my business acumen

Now that you have a better understanding of the 'why', here are some ways you could find a mentor(s):

- *Through applying to a formal programme* – there are lots of initiatives and programmes (mentoring programmes, but also programmes such as the NHS CEP which provides a mentor as part of the process) out there; you just need to have a look and take the plunge to apply.

- *By being proactive* – try asking senior colleagues (and your peers) if they would support you. You may want to look for those who are interested in teaching, or who have a history of mentoring others. Carefully consider their careers or areas of interest and see if this aligns with what you need help with.

- *Attending events* – as above, you should try to network within (and of course outside of) your organisation. Try to build a professional relationship over time. Once you have made some connections, you may want to ask if they would consider mentoring you. It might seem daunting but think of the benefits if they say yes!

Now let's look at a few steps you can take to approach a mentor.

Depending on the format of mentoring, i.e. a formal or more informal style, your approach may differ (you may choose to speak to them in person or send them an email or direct message). However, there are some commonalities in *how* you can effectively approach someone that we will look at below:

- *Be clear on your why* – depending on the situation (i.e. through a platform designed to 'match' you to a mentor or a work colleague) you may want to send them an introductory email about *who you are* and the *specific* help you needed. Be as clear as possible, especially if the person knows very little about you and your background.

- *Explain why you chose to contact them* instead of someone else in the same field or workplace, or with the same skill set and experience. This might be because of their extensive experience or their demonstrated track record of supporting others, or because their values and beliefs align with yours.

- *Think about whether you want to directly or indirectly ask them to mentor you.* This clearly does not apply if you are part of a formal programme where mentoring is what you are expecting / have been promised. However, if you are trying to establish a more informal mentoring relationship you might want to consider if the question "will you be my mentor?" is the right one. Sometimes mentoring relationships are not explicitly labelled as this (although they clearly are!) and it might be offputting, especially if someone does not know exactly what this entails. If you do ask this question then ensure you follow up with what this means to you – i.e. general advice and guidance, emotional support or a more assertive approach in helping you achieve your goals. You should also include how much time you expect the mentor to dedicate to you; for example, perhaps meeting once a month or every quarter could be sufficient.

> **Example 3.4 – How I have approached mentors**
>
> Let's look at formal mentoring first. Depending on the programme you are part of, you might be matched with one mentor by the programme or you may have to choose a mentor yourself out of a 'pool' of mentors. Usually, the mentors identified will be based on some similarities and the help you specifically need. With one experience, I was initially helped with the selection based on my needs, but I then had to justify why I selected that particular mentor before they would agree to mentor me. In less formal situations I have simply struck up a conversation with someone who I feel has the expertise or role I am interested in and asked to book a meeting with them. I usually ask to hear more about their story and background first, which helps me determine if this could be a successful mentoring relationship for both of us.

3.6.3   Maintaining a successful mentoring arrangement

To maintain a successful mentoring relationship, you of course need participation from both parties. You could use some elements of the 'manage-up' approach, which would include:

- *Completing a self-assessment* – write down what you need help with and how your potential mentor could help you with this. This will ensure clarity for both parties from the start.
- *Effective time management* – set a clear plan for what you would like to achieve during the meeting(s) with your mentor and create a plan of action. Discussing both your communication styles and preferences is imperative not only to make the best use of time but also for the success of the mentoring relationship.
- *Put the work in* – ensure you complete actions (if possible) between meetings and continuously assess how the relationship

is progressing. Sending updates about your progress might be helpful. Try to ensure there aren't large gaps between meetings as this might hinder your progress and the relationship you have with your mentor.

> I aim to meet my NHS CEP mentor monthly (which does happen). My mentor sets me a task to complete between meetings and I usually select one or two key takeaways from our session. He also asks me what I would like help with each session, so it is more self-directed and meaningful.

Finally, some additional tips for working with your mentor include the following:

- Show your mentor that you are thankful for their help, which could be via a thank you card or offering to buy them a coffee.
- Consider asking them if you can help them in some way. For example, if they are writing a book you could send them some useful resources for reading. Remember, the relationship should be positive and beneficial for you both.
- Think about agreeing a set time period for mentoring, such as 3–6 months. This is not compulsory, especially if it is informal. You both may continue the mentoring relationship beyond this time so don't worry that it is always set in stone.
- Whilst there are many benefits to mentoring, there can also be negatives. So assess the mentor–mentee relationship for both parties frequently, and decide whether it is favourable to continue.

Example 3.5

During one of the sessions with my mentor through the Emerging Women Leader's Programme I asked if they needed help of any kind. They said that I might be useful in reviewing a new document they were constructing for patients and my experience as a GP would be useful. They also asked me to share the document with my colleagues to see if they also had any feedback.

In *Chapter 4* you can start categorising your portfolio of activities with practical templates.

Chapter summary

- Career success is much more than financial reward and seniority. It can be divided into objective factors, which include salary, position and promotions, and subjective factors, which include job satisfaction, fulfilment and achievement. You need to work out what success means to you personally.
- There are three types of mobility required for the journey towards career success: upward mobility (movement up a theoretical hierarchical ladder), sponsored mobility (when someone is supported by a more powerful or elite individual or organisation) and contest mobility (when success is based solely on an individual's own efforts).
- The two main predictors of success are human capital (which includes social capital; a person's network of contacts) and organisational sponsorship (the support from colleagues, and training and resources offered).
  - It is important to understand our own social capital and how we can maximise the impact of existing social networks to achieve our goals, whilst fostering new connections which will positively affect our chances of success in our chosen field. The '4 Ps' to excellent networking are preparation, projection, participation and progress.
  - Organisational sponsorship covers the support given to an individual by their employer, and also the concept of mentoring, where an experienced professional gives support and advice over a long period of time. Both can increase the chances of career success, and effort should be made to find and approach multiple mentors from a variety of sources.
- Particular character traits (neuroticism, conscientiousness, extroversion, agreeableness, and openness to experience) are also predictors of success. Whatever our characteristics, being proactive when it comes to networking and our career, will reap rewards.
- Additional qualifications contribute to an individual's human capital, as does their length of experience in a particular role. Many skills, such as leadership and problem-solving, will be transferable throughout your career.
- Career planning is essential at the start of the journey to career success, and can be achieved through coaching, counselling or self-help guides. Readiness for career planning involves a high awareness of your own circumstances, characteristics and requirement for support.

Chapter 4:
A practical template for creating your career

By the end of this chapter you should be able to:

- Understand what categorising a portfolio is, why it is important and how you can categorise your own career
- Think about exactly what is needed for each activity in your portfolio
- Select a few key ways to get started with creating your career
- Describe some basic strategies for managing your time and workload
- Set some SMART goals.

4.1 Categorising your portfolio

4.1.1 The importance of categorising your activities

As I mentioned in *Chapter 1* (and as you will see later on in *Chapter 6*), portfolio careers take years to develop and refine. I have learnt to continually place my portfolio of activities (which includes paid and unpaid work) into categories (or the types of work I do). This is not only helpful to me when I think about the variety of work I do (and what I want to do in the future), but it also helps others (potential employers, peers and colleagues) understand what my portfolio career encompasses.

Categories can be divided up as you see fit; it really depends on how much detail you feel will be useful for you. I would try to start with it kept simple and broad; for example, you might divide your portfolio into general practice, medical writing and public speaking, with general practice as your main career. Having one main career with additional satellite careers is known as 'anchoring' (see *Figure 4.1*) or 'one dominant career anchor' as detailed in the 'career anchor model':

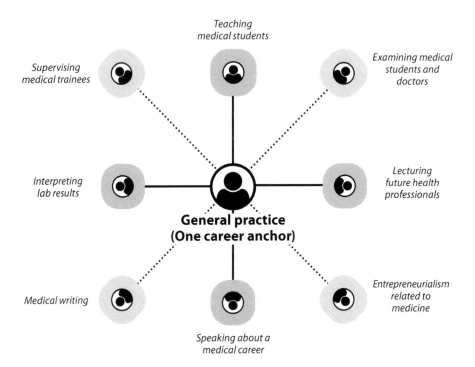

Figure 4.1 *'Anchoring' describes having one main career with additional satellite careers.*

Alternatively, you might prefer to have multiple career anchors (see *Figure 4.2*). You may choose to divide your work into clinical and non-clinical roles, and then further subdivide each of these roles. For example, you could further subdivide general practice (especially if you want to focus on a portfolio career within general practice):

- NHS and private work
- Salaried and self-employed work
- Face-to-face consultations and remote work / teleconsulting
- Practical procedures such as joint injections and minor surgeries.

I have provided you with a template in the next section to help you categorise your career, but do feel free to develop your own templates and include as much (or as little) detail as you like.

> Remember that this is not meant to be rigid – your portfolio of activities might change depending on your financial situation, personal satisfaction or life events.

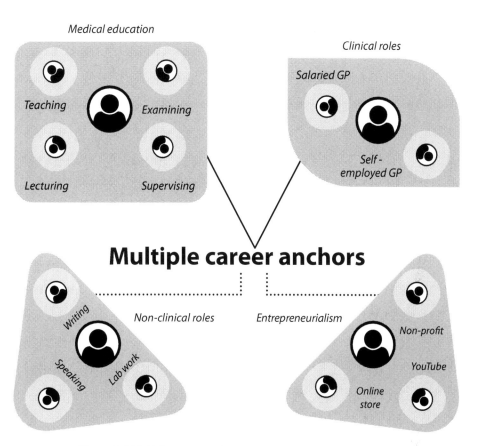

Figure 4.2 *Multiple career anchors.*

Think about how your personality traits impact the way you categorise your portfolio activities.

- If you fit into the 'openness' personality trait you are more open to new experiences and trying new things, and so might decide to have multiple career anchors, especially if you are creative too.

- This might also be the case if you are more 'extroverted' and so enjoy meeting new people and having a wide array of interests and activities.

- If you are more 'conscientious' on the other hand, you might prefer to be extremely organised in planning out your portfolio activities and enjoy having a regular routine and structure to your working week. For you, having one dominant career anchor and slowly adding in satellite careers as you progress is likely to be better.

4.1.2 How to categorise your portfolio

Before we look at the process of categorising, let's draw together what you learnt in the preceding chapters about yourself and how the wider environment affects the development of your career. This will help you when it comes to deciding what goes into each category of your career.

By the end of *Chapter 2*, you developed a better understanding of who you are and what potential jobs you might be suited to – now would be a good time to quickly review your top three interests, values and beliefs and skills and qualities (see the end of *Section 2.4*). Also look at the possible careers you matched your interests to (*Section 2.4.1*) and why you thought they would be suitable (or unsuitable). Did you note down any wider environmental factors that could potentially impact your career now and in the future?

In *Chapter 3* you started to decide what career success means to you. Review the table you created in *Section 3.2.1* where you looked at important subjective and objective factors, such as personal satisfaction at work and financial rewards. You should also have a clear understanding of your personality type; if not, then completing the 'Big Five' questionnaire now would be helpful (see *Section 3.2.3*). Finally, we worked through the RIASEC Hexagon to discern what type of working environment might suit you based on your personality type (see *Section 3.4.2*).

Use a table to bring all this information together; with everything in one place we can start to categorise your portfolio (*I have provided a few examples*):

Your top three	Personality type	Portfolio activity	Contributing factors (wider environment)
Interests - Clinical practice - Medical education - Arts and crafts	Big Five – scored highly in: - Conscientiousness - Extroversion - Openness to experience	A combination of GP NHS and private face-to-face and remote work – because sometimes I enjoy interacting with others but at times I prefer to problem-solve independently I'd like to teach GP trainees and become an appraiser – but I am not sure what my options are (courses?)	Family – it can be hard to take care of two children whilst working full-time; enlisting more help from family and friends might help me develop my career Finances – I would have to save or look for funding to develop a business making clothes / painting. Any courses might be funded by HEE or my practice for teaching opportunities

Your top three	Personality type	Portfolio activity	Contributing factors (wider environment)
		I want to develop my artistic side more and turn this into a potential business but not sure how to get started	The current economic / political environment, e.g. cost of living might mean that my portfolio career plan might take a little longer to implement
Values and beliefs - Being authentic - Staying true to who I am - Honesty and integrity	RIASEC Hexagon: - Social – I prefer interacting with others - Investigative – I enjoy solving difficult problems and at times prefer this to interacting with others - I am artistic – I love making new art such as painting, knitting and making clothes		
Skills and qualities - Strong-minded - Highly organised - Compassionate	Cognitive information pyramid: - I need to look more closely at how I make decisions to avoid making similar future mistakes and knowing what options are open to me		

We will look at specific areas (such as the level of investment needed for your activity) and how you can think about acquiring them for your portfolio career. Before we do that, however, you will need to categorise (but not necessarily compartmentalise) your activities.

> You will find that some of your activities cannot be compartmentalised, such that they cannot be completely separated. For example, my portfolio career, whilst in 'neat' categories, is all tied to my clinical work in some capacity. Lecturing requires me to have clinical experience, and so whilst they fit into clinical work or general practice and medical education, they are inextricably linked.

Categorising is particularly useful if you have some portfolio activities but do not have a structure or a clear idea of what you are currently doing and what you might have additional time for. Or, you may not have started yet, so the template below will help you to clarify exactly what you would like to do in the future.

Figure 4.3 is an example of my portfolio at one point in time (the categories have remained broadly the same despite changing some of the activities themselves).

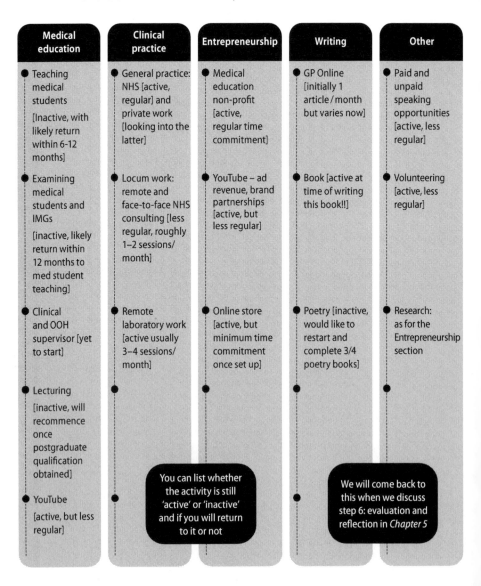

Medical education	Clinical practice	Entrepreneurship	Writing	Other
Teaching medical students [Inactive, with likely return within 6-12 months]	General practice: NHS [active, regular] and private work [looking into the latter]	Medical education non-profit [active, regular time commitment]	GP Online [initially 1 article/month but varies now]	Paid and unpaid speaking opportunities [active, less regular]
Examining medical students and IMGs [inactive, likely return within 12 months to med student teaching]	Locum work: remote and face-to-face NHS consulting [less regular, roughly 1–2 sessions/month]	YouTube – ad revenue, brand partnerships [active, but less regular]	Book [active at time of writing this book!!]	Volunteering [active, less regular]
Clinical and OOH supervisor [yet to start]	Remote laboratory work [active usually 3–4 sessions/month]	Online store [active, but minimum time commitment once set up]	Poetry [inactive, would like to restart and complete 3/4 poetry books]	Research: as for the Entrepreneurship section
Lecturing [inactive, will recommence once postgraduate qualification obtained]		You can list whether the activity is still 'active' or 'inactive' and if you will return to it or not		We will come back to this when we discuss step 6: evaluation and reflection in *Chapter 5*
YouTube [active, but less regular]				

Figure 4.3 *Categorising your portfolio.*

Whether you have an existing (but perhaps basic) portfolio or are in the process of creating a completely new one, you can use the next set of templates to:

- List *the activity* or describe exactly what it involves (if future activity)
- The *skills and qualities* it requires (or the ones you use currently and how you can improve them)
- The current level of *investment* or the investment needed (future activity) and the potential returns on investment (both current and future activities)
- Your *enjoyment* level (if a current activity)
- How much of a *priority* this is in your career / life (can list for both current and future activities).

Let's start with any existing portfolio activities you may have (I've added an example to get you started):

Activity	How can you further enhance your skill set / qualities?	What investment does this require?	Potential returns on investment	How much, on a scale of 1–10, do I enjoy this activity now? What could affect this?
Teaching medical students	Further understanding of medical education theory through a postgraduate qualification in medical education or the like	Time – c. 1 day per week for study Cost – can apply for funding from HEE but may require £9k per year	Will improve my knowledge and thus improve the quality of teaching I provide May lead to further opportunities, e.g. designing exams / working as a lecturer at the medical school, which will be an additional viable income stream	8/10 – if preparation time increases or clinical work encroaches on time for teaching

Future portfolio activities:

Use the activities in the table you created above (at the start of *Section 4.1.2*) as a starting point. We will then set some SMART goals in *Section 4.4* to help make them become a reality.

Let's move on to future portfolio activities (I've added an example to get you started):

Activity	What does it involve?	What skills and qualities do you need for this activity?	How can you further enhance your skill set / qualities?	What investment will this require?	Potential returns on investment	What is the priority?
Occupational health physician	Assessing and supporting employees in the workplace; ensuring they are safe both mentally / physically at work Good work–life balance with 9–5 days Writing reports	Skills include problem-solving, working independently more frequently, time management, excellent communication Qualities include patience, emotional intelligence, conflict resolution	Diploma in Occupational Health Networking and speaking to those in the field	Time – 2 weeks, for online / face-to-face course; 50 hours for portfolio; 50 hours for revision and exams Cost – £2–3k	Better work–life balance Can be lucrative and another income stream Options for ways of working; can sub-specialise	Ideally I would like to make a start, i.e. book within the next 2 years, after some other projects and commitments

Activity	What does it involve?	What skills and qualities do you need for this activity?	How can you further enhance your skill set / qualities?	What investment will this require?	Potential returns on investment	What is the priority?

4.2 How to actually get started, including some financial and legal aspects to consider

You might be thinking, OK I now know what types of activities I want to include in my portfolio career, but how do I structure my current working situation to help incorporate or even replace some existing areas in my career?

> *Sometimes the hardest thing is to start, but if you don't start you won't know if you will succeed or not. Remember, if you fail, that is OK. However, it is important you learn from your failure. Perhaps it may not even be a failure, more of a redirection on a different path. As we learnt in Chapter 3, how you think and feel determines your behaviour, so try to think positively.*

4.2.1 Deciding on how you want to structure your portfolio career

You might not be sure how to realistically get started with your portfolio career, so here are a few options to consider:

1. *Using your spare time – during evenings, weekends, annual and study leave –* just as I was getting started with developing my portfolio career I signed up to full-time GP training. It definitely slowed the pace down, but I spent a lot of my free time working on the areas I was passionate about. It was hard but I made it work and it ultimately helped me to become a better doctor. For example, my work delivering courses to schools took place largely during my evenings, weekends and annual leave. Writing for GP Online occurred when I had a free moment, which again would likely be weekends when I was more relaxed and had the time and space to be creative. Another example might be if you are considering starting a career in aesthetics. If you pair up with a beauty salon to offer your services, your busiest time might be weekends. Such an option may be temporary, but because you are just starting out it can help you to decide what works and what does not.

2. *Reducing your hours – working part-time, taking time out of training or a sabbatical.* Working part-time is an option but this might be difficult if it results in a salary reduction (unless your activity can make up for any financial losses) and it could make the overall training pathway harder (due to lack of continuity, for example) and longer (from three to five years, potentially). Once qualified

as a GP you can take one or two years out of clinical work (you would need to re-train if longer than this). You might want to think about how you can still earn an income as clinical work (such as locuming) would not be an option if taking a sabbatical. If you are a trainee, you could apply for an Out of Programme (OOP) experience, although this does need approval from your postgraduate dean and possibly the Royal College or faculty you are part of.

3. *Leaving completely* – leaving your current form of employment and leaping into another opportunity (or opportunities). This might be the 'riskiest' option but if you feel this is best for you and would enable the fastest growth, then why not give it a go? Create a plan (and a back-up plan or two!) for how this could work.

4.2.2 The financial and legal implications of a portfolio career

Other considerations when structuring your portfolio would be your form of employment. In this section we'll look at some of the ways you can do this: basically you'll be choosing between conventional employment and being self-employed.

So let's start by considering the options available to you:

- One main employed role with multiple self-employed or freelance roles as supplementary incomes (think back to *Section 4.1* – one main career anchor with additional satellite careers). This could include seasonal work such as examining medical students or delivering exam courses (which is a somewhat less secure form of employment).

- Multiple part-time employed roles (this could be seen as multiple career anchors, as seen in *Section 4.1*). One issue of having more than one *employed* role at a time, is that if you want to request annual leave it might be trickier to coordinate across the various roles. Since this can be a problem (it was for me), one secure form of employment may be preferable; for me this was NHS general practice work (salaried, part-time role) and having a combination of freelance part-time roles to supplement this income and also to fuel my passions which I could not do without.

- Mainly self-employed work (perhaps as a GP partner or locum GP).

Now let's look now at some of the financial and legal considerations to the ways in which you can work. Some of this was covered briefly in *Chapter 1* when we looked at the various ways you can work as a GP.

Employed vs. self-employed work

Some of the main considerations are set out below, whether you decide to work as an employee or as someone who is self-employed, either as a sole trader or through a limited company.

Here are some features of working in either way:

Self-employed (sole trader / limited company (Ltd))	Employed
Easy to set up – register with His Majesty's Revenue and Customs (HMRC) as self-employed and/or Companies House if setting up a limited company.	No set-up required.
You can still make pension contributions, for example if you are locuming, but would need to complete the necessary forms for Primary Care Support England (PCSE). However, some companies do pay pension contributions even if you are self-employed.	Pension contributions will be deducted directly from your salary, and your employer also contributes towards your pension.
There is some additional paperwork to complete such as submitting a self-assessment form to HMRC for each tax year, or preparing annual accounts for a limited company.	No additional paperwork to complete.
You are personally liable for any financial and legal issues that arise as a sole trader. However, this does not apply if registered as a limited company.	No personal liability.
You can deduct expenses such as uniform, travel costs and lunch, which might reduce the amount of tax you have to pay.	Does not apply.

Self-employed (sole trader / limited company (Ltd))	Employed
You keep your profits as a sole trader. However, if you are working with others you may have to share any profits you make through the limited company (other directors, investors or shareholders), unless you set up a limited company on your own, of course. Depending how much you make, you might want to consider setting up a limited company which might make it more cost-effective (see below).	Does not apply.
You can hire a contractor to complete work for you – e.g. video editing, marketing or admin work – if you are registered as either a sole trader or limited company. You can register as an employer instead. However, this comes with additional considerations such as insurance, salaries, setting up employment contracts and employee rights.	Does not apply.
Depending on how much you make and how long you have been operating for, it might be more difficult to secure a mortgage.	It might be easier to secure a mortgage, as work is meant to be more secure and especially as your salary would not be expected to fluctuate like it could when working as someone who is self-employed (potentially).

Here are some additional pointers:

- Profits:
  - If you are earning over c. £40 000 per annum it might be worth setting up a limited company. The positives to this would be that you could pay yourself a lower salary each year, such as around £700/month (this would be below the threshold of National Insurance contributions but would not affect your

benefits) and pay yourself dividends. This might include more paperwork, though, such as completing a self-assessment tax return for dividends (which you would have to complete anyway if you were a sole trader).

- Paying tax:
  - You also have to consider the various types of tax, such as corporation tax, that you would have to pay if you set up as a limited company (it might actually work out better for you than if you were a sole trader, as the rate of corporation tax is usually lower than the higher rates of income tax).

- Privacy:
  - If setting up a limited company you would need to register on Companies House, which can be accessed by the public (this does not take long, but you would need a registered address). You can dissolve the company if needs be (again this is not a complicated process).

Overall, it mainly depends on how much you see yourself making. You might start off as self-employed and if your career progresses, you could set up a limited company.

Limited liability partnership or LLP

This is similar to working via a limited company, but those in the partnership (i.e. the members), although under one umbrella, essentially operate as separate entities. This means the members in the LLP are legally separate from the partnership itself (and therefore not liable for any debts that could occur, similar to a limited company) and do not have to pay corporation tax both on profits and also on salaries, on dividends to directors and/or shareholders (unlike a limited company). The LLP generally has more flexibility on how it can run, as it is not confined to Companies Act 2006 (like a limited company is).

Some drawbacks include requiring a minimum of two members, whereas you can set up a limited company (or register as a sole trader) on your own, having to share financial accounts with Companies House which is public, and potentially more financial costs due to administration and reporting costs.

If you want to consider becoming a sole trader or setting up a limited company (or LLP) then my advice would be to hire an accountant, which does save you time and potentially money. As you will see from the rest of this section, there is a lot to think about and you might prefer focusing on other matters instead.

Accountants can submit the necessary paperwork to HMRC and may speak on your behalf if there are any issues that arise. Whether you choose a medical or non-medical accountant depends on the work you are doing (and how cost-effective they are). I personally have a non-medical accountant and complete the end of year pensions certificate myself (which some GPs pay their medical accountants to do).

4.3 Time management and balancing workload (including how to stay sane!)

Rather than providing you with cliché tips on time management and productivity, I hope that this section provides you with a few key pointers that have helped me on my own journey as a portfolio GP.

Take on one project or portfolio activity at a time

It makes sense that it might be hard to dedicate enough time and produce high-quality or favourable outcomes if you are spread too thin; this is something that all portfolio GPs have to consider. It can be tempting to want to do it all, but that can lead to burnout and not actually achieving anything. Think about committing to one or two projects (such as a diploma or monthly newsletter) at a time. Once those are completed you can then think about moving on to something else; you might also find that some of your portfolio activities naturally become phased out over time. Being able to juggle multiple projects is an art, but with unexpected life events such as illness or bereavement it can sometimes be unachievable. Be realistic and focus initially on one or two portfolio activities simultaneously; if you can do more than this, then great, but think seriously about what is achievable based on your current personal and work commitments.

Don't say yes to every opportunity because it sounds good

Following on from the above point, try not to get caught up in wearing multiple hats simply because this looks impressive or the opportunity sounds really exciting. Be strategic in the creation of your portfolio career and carve it out wisely. Of course, you can sign up to things for fun, but if you are thinking about developing a portfolio career, only say yes to the opportunities that are going to steer you in the right direction.

It is OK if your timeline changes – don't always be too focused on rigid deadlines

The deadline for completing the writing of this book was one year, but here I am in my second year of trying to complete it! But that's OK – I have had a lot of work and family commitments that I have had to prioritise and sometimes that happens. Often we get very focused on meeting our deadlines and, whilst focusing and setting targets is important, it is equally important to realise when we need to push deadlines back and not be too hard on ourselves. Be flexible with your deadlines and realise that you will get there, even if it takes a little longer than you anticipated.

Use chunks of time wisely

Every week, like most people, I have a routine with a clear structure of what I must complete. As you can imagine, this is mostly work and family commitments – lecturing, clinical work, shopping, cooking, cleaning, etc. Anything else such as writing articles, creating content and filming YouTube videos is a nice part of my portfolio career, but it is not compulsory. When I do aim to integrate these activities into my working week or month, I tend to think about how these additional 'nice to have' activities can fit into my main schedule. Will this task take roughly 30 minutes or 1 hour? Can I do it in 10 minutes? Examples would be setting aside 2 hours to edit a YouTube video or 20 minutes to review some work at Medschool Xtra. The same can be applied to work / life commitments, such as completing forms or reviewing my accounts. If I have a spare 30 minutes, I think, what would I be able to do in this time?

Another tactic I use is thinking about the activity before I sit down to complete it. When I was at school, my science teacher explained to the class that before attempting any questions in our exam papers, it was a good idea to flick through the questions and let your brain start thinking about the possible answers, subconsciously. An example of how I use this today is when it came to editing this chapter. I was asked to write this section about time management. I started to use small blocks of time to think about the points I would write. It would be at the back of my mind, so my brain was working away, thinking about what I could write. I use a similar tactic when structuring an article, scripting a YouTube video or even writing a poem. I might make some handwritten bullet points or short notes on my phone. When I sit down to complete the task, i.e. write this section or an article, it takes much less time than if I hadn't thought about it over the preceding week(s).

Lean on your support network (and support your network too!)

People often ask me "how are you able to do everything you do?" Or comments are made such as "you are doing so much!". The truth is I wouldn't be able to do anything if it were not for those around me. My parents and brother support my husband and me with childcare commitments, which means we can work more and save on childcare, and enables us to spend some quality time together. As we learnt in *Section 3.5.2*, networks or relationships are a two-way street, so always think about how you can give and not just take. Asking for and accepting help is crucial to staying sane, avoiding burnout and achieving your goals.

4.4 Goal setting

To make your career a reality you will need to be *intentional*, which partly means creating a clear plan. Writing out your plan in succinct steps is crucial to ensuring your career becomes a reality (but allow some room for flexibility too).

If you already have a portfolio career but want more clarity or a new direction, this is the perfect time to stop, review and create a new (or revised) plan of action. Next, we will look at making that plan work, specifically:

- how you can create Specific, Measurable, Achievable, Relevant and Timely (SMART) goals
- some issues with goal setting and how you can overcome these.

You should now have categorised your portfolio and listed portfolio activities in more detail; so now it is time to work through each activity and create a SMART goal. You may want to be selective with which activities you want to focus on first and therefore the goals you create – start by selecting one or two to begin with.

You may have set some SMART goals before, so take a moment to think carefully about how you can create clearer goals using this method. If you haven't written SMART goals previously, they can help you to achieve your overall goal by setting much smaller steps to take. Then you regularly evaluate progress and adjust the goal as you achieve the different steps needed. An example is shown in *Figure 4.4:*

SPECIFIC

Teaching medical students

Do your research so you can be as clear as possible about what you would like to achieve. What steps do you need to take to make it happen?

| To obtain a teaching qualification | ➡ | I will research the entry requirements and fees |

⬇

| To obtain a Masters in medical education | ➡ | I will apply for funding and save |

⬇

| To obtain a Masters in medical education from UCL | ➡ | I will set aside time each week to complete the application form |

MEASURABLE

Teaching medical students

How can you ensure you are on track to meet your outcomes?

| One month before starting to achieve my goal I would have made a list of entry requirements, fees and applied for funding | ➡ | I will complete one section of the application form each week and track my progress with 'x' application weekly |

ACHIEVABLE

Teaching medical students

Can you realistically achieve this goal? What evidence base do you have for this? What resources do you have or need?

I have taught medical students for several years and gained lots of positive feedback

I have completed a module at Masters level achieving MERIT

I can incorporate the learning within my working week, occasional weekends and study leave

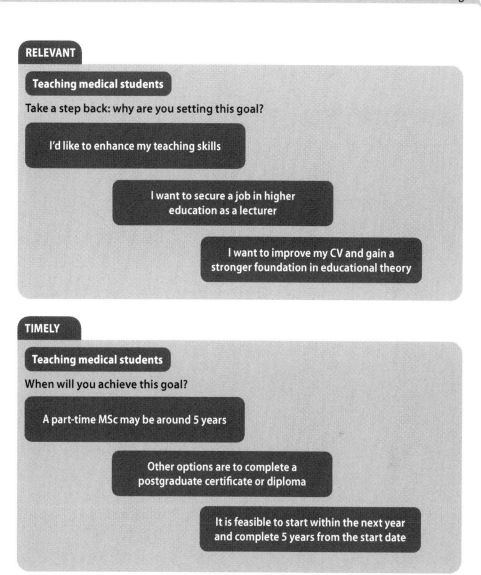

Figure 4.4 *An example of SMART goals relating to teaching medical students.*

Use the template below to create three to five SMART goals (you can start with one or two portfolio activities initially which you would have created at the start of this chapter):

Specific	What exactly do you want to achieve?
Measurable	How will you keep track of whether you are on target?
Achievable	How will you ensure that your goal is within reach?
Relevant	Why are you setting this goal?
Timely	When will you achieve this goal?

Finally, a few points on setting goals. As outlined in the book *Atomic Habits* by James Clear, focusing on your systems or processes (how you achieve your goals and the direction you want to go in) is much better than focusing solely on your goals (the end results or what you want to achieve). Here are a few reasons why it is better to set identity-based habits than outcome-based habits:

1. The goal becomes the sole focus and can affect your happiness

When you set goals, the end point or goal becomes your focus instead of the right *systems* you need to have in place. Good systems and processes, not the goal, helps differentiate those who 'win' and those who don't, even though they may have had the exact same goal.

2. Goals last for a moment; long-term progress is what you need

What happens when you achieve your goal? Where do you go next? You might feel despondent when you have achieved your goal and you're not sure what direction you need to go in next. James Clear suggests that for many, after a specific goal is achieved, problematic systems and behaviours reappear. An example he gives is setting the goal of keeping your room tidy, which might be something you find really hard to do. Once you tidy your room, you achieve your goal and might feel happy for that moment. But how do you *maintain* a tidy room? How do you address the issues that prevent you from keeping your room tidy? You can apply this to other examples, such as someone who wants to lose weight; if they do not implement the right systems it would be very easy after they have lost a set amount of weight to put the weight straight back on.

So, how can you achieve long-lasting results? Let's look at an example relating to portfolio careers. You want to create a portfolio career, right? OK, but let's re-word this. Let's look at the goal of you wanting to *become a portfolio GP or someone with a portfolio career.* This changes the goal from outcome to identity-based and thus will have longer-lasting results. Your identity is a combination of what you believe and your values. *So, how would someone behave and act if they were a portfolio GP?*

Let's make this even more specific. One aspect of my portfolio career is writing. I wanted to write poetry as I really enjoyed this and found it therapeutic. I also wanted to write opinion-based and factual pieces for medical publications. I also really wanted to write a book. Whilst these were goals, I did not focus too much on the outcomes and instead I focused *more on the writing itself* – becoming *a writer and author.* I focused on the systems and processes that would help me achieve those goals. Early on in my writing career I asked an editor for advice on securing a long-term writing role. The advice was simply to "keep on writing". I was unsure how that advice would really help me, because I was hoping I would be pointed in the direction of where to apply or submit more articles to. However, I kept writing and without knowing it I *became* a writer *and* secured a long-term role at GP Online. I also self-published a poetry book and, of course, you are reading my book about portfolio careers!

So, whilst goal setting and doing it well are important, try not to focus too much on the final outcome – focus instead on the journey, the processes and how these will change you as a person.

Chapter summary

- Categorising your activities involves thinking about the variety of work that you do; this should be in light of what you learnt about yourself and your personality type in *Chapter 2* and what career success means to you in *Chapter 3*.
- Using the categorising template will help you to clarify what you would like to do in the future.
- With any potential future portfolio activity, consideration will need to be given to finding out what is involved, what skills and qualities the activity requires, what investment of time and/or money may be required to realise it, and what the potential benefits are.
- Getting started on your portfolio career will require changes to the way you manage your time; this will need to be balanced with the potential for faster growth.
- Creating and maintaining a portfolio career is an art that requires some innovative thinking about how you can balance everything successfully.
- Forms of employment vary, but the main choice is between conventional employment and being self-employed. These can be combined in numerous ways; each with their own financial considerations and benefits.
- If you choose the self-employed route, the options are as a sole trader or through a limited company or limited liability partnership.
- The temptation to take on too many projects should be resisted, to avoid over-commitment and burnout; time is precious and should be used wisely.
- SMART goals can be used to help you assess progress towards the portfolio activities you wish to pursue. Regular evaluation of the goals is important.
- Aiming for long-term, process-based progress is better than specific goals being your sole focus. The journey towards the goal, focusing on who you want to become is, I would argue, more important than setting the goal.

Chapter 5:
Evaluating (and re-evaluating) your career

> **By the end of this chapter you should be able to:**
> - Understand the importance of evaluating your career
> - Accurately evaluate your career
> - Think about diversifying your career as a more experienced GP.

5.1 The importance of evaluating your career

Stopping to evaluate your career at certain points (whether forced to or not) is imperative not only to your career success but also to your mental and physical wellbeing – even small changes to your career journey can have a big impact.

In the preceding chapters we have considered the most important factors that will enable you to create a portfolio career. We have looked at your personality and any environmental aspects that may affect your career (see *Chapter 2*) and at the importance of understanding what career success means to you to ensure you are always on *your* road to success (*Chapter 3*). In *Chapter 4* we applied a lot of this information to specific portfolio activities that you can now start to develop.

An important element to creating a successful and sustainable portfolio career is to regularly review all this information and make essential changes (however small). It has taken you a lot of time and effort to compile this information, so it is important not to waste it!

5.2 How to accurately evaluate your career

In this section we will look at the various methods that you can use to evaluate and re-evaluate where you are on your career journey.

Evaluation is defined as 'the process of *judging* or *calculating* the *quality, importance, amount* or *value* of something'. Re-evaluating is repeating this process again and again as required. It is good practice to set specific timeframes on such evaluation / re-evaluation, whether quarterly, annually or when you reach a milestone in your career. Being proactive, and acting before you

feel dissatisfied or something goes wrong in your career, is always
advisable.

5.2.1   Five steps to evaluate your career

Let's now look at five steps you can use to critically evaluate your
portfolio career on a regular basis:

Step 1 – where are you now?

- Use the table of portfolio activities you created in *Section 4.1.2* to
  look at your current portfolio activities. Go through each activity
  and update with any changes where necessary. Consider how
  long ago you last reviewed this table and whether it is all still
  relevant.

Step 2 – what has worked well?

- What do you think has gone well with each activity? Consider
  why this might be. Be specific – you might want to revisit the
  SMART goals you created in *Section 4.4* to determine if you
  achieved them. Try to list four positives for each activity and/or
  SMART goal you created. It is important to focus on the positives
  and to do this *first*. Remember (*Section 3.4.3*) that it is too easy to
  focus on the negative first instead of highlighting what we did
  well.

Step 3 – what has not worked so well?

- Consider what has not worked so well, but focus on the reasons
  why things haven't worked out in the way you hoped.

Step 4 – what can you change?

- If things did not go to plan, what have you learnt from the reasons
  why they didn't work so well, so that you can make adjustments
  so this does not happen again? If you are happy with your
  progress, is there anything you need to do to continue on this
  trajectory?

Step 5 – where do you want to be?

- Finally, where would you like to be in the near and distant future?
  What will your career look like in two, five or even ten years from
  now? You may not want to think so far ahead, but use timelines
  as a guide to ensure that you continue to re-evaluate.

Complete the table overleaf to help evaluate your portfolio activities. Use this to evaluate one portfolio activity and/or SMART goal (*I have provided an example to help*):

Where are you now?	What has worked well?	What has not worked well?	What can you change (and when)?	Where do you want to be?
Lecturing medical students	Transitioned from working 1 to 3 days a week	Not enough active learning strategies used (mentioned during student feedback)	Research more strategies to improve student experience	Working towards being a course lead for this course or another at the university
	Promoted to module lead	Need to work on my time management when at work	Speak to my line manager to see what can be done to help me manage my time better. Think about the way I prepare my lectures – is there anything I can remove or change?	My SMART goal is...
	Working towards my PG Cert (funded by the university)			
	(you also need to think about why these things have gone well; see Section 5.2.2 next for help)			

Now use this space to complete your own evaluation of your portfolio activities.

Where are you now?	What has worked well?	What has not worked well?	What can you change (and when)?	Where do you want to be?

5.2.2   SWOT analysis and the G-Star model

SWOT (Strengths, Weaknesses, Opportunities and Threats) analysis

Although originating in business and traditionally applied at an organisational level, the SWOT analysis can also be applied to individuals. It helps you to:

- clearly understand what you can offer to others – Strengths
- understand what you may need to improve upon – Weaknesses
- identify what gaps in the market you may be well-qualified to fill, by looking at what your peers may or may not be doing – Opportunities
- evaluate what challenges you face, such as competitors in your field / the field you want to enter into – Threats.

Whilst there are always limitations, the analysis can be used regularly at set points along your career trajectory.

A SWOT analysis can be used *alongside* the five-step process from *Section 5.2.1,* from step 2 to step 4:

- Step 2 – what has worked well? – your Strengths
- Step 3 – what has not worked so well? – your Weaknesses
- Step 4 – what can you change? – your Opportunities and Threats.

Step 2 – what has worked well?

Continuing to use the 'lecturing medical students' activity as an example:

- What went well:
  - I have transitioned from working for one day a week to three days a week
  - I have been promoted to module lead.

- Why it went well:
  - Good organisational skills which helped with lesson planning
  - Use of initiative and innovative thinking when designing and writing assessments
  - Excellent feedback from staff and students.

Step 3 – what has not worked so well?

Repeat the process here, including the 'why' and 'what' you can do to overcome these weaknesses.

Step 4 – what can you change?

Here you can assess what opportunities are available for you in the future. Are you good at seeking opportunities out? Does the practice support your development as a medical educator? Perhaps you are teaching medical students, but you'd like to teach FY2 doctors or GP trainees; what opportunities are available at your practice or elsewhere? Are any of your colleagues working in academia, such as at a university? If so, perhaps there is an opportunity to use them as an inspiration or see where there are gaps in that field that you can fill – maybe in research or teaching methods?

Also consider what potential threats exist. Do you have 'protected' time to teach medical students? Is the time taken to prepare for the sessions encroaching upon your work–life balance? What are your peers doing – could they pose a threat, perhaps to your chance of getting a new job if they are also applying, or might they be starting a research project in the same area as you?

The G-Star model

This is a tool traditionally used for mentoring, but it can also be used to encourage you to think about where you are on your journey and a particular obstacle(s) you might be facing. If you do have a mentor, it can be used to help facilitate mentoring discussions and provide your mentor with an insight into the challenges you want to address. The G-Star acronym stands for:

- What are your **G**oals?
- What **S**ituation are you facing?
- What is your **T**hinking currently?
- What **A**ctions are you considering?
- What **R**esults do you expect?

And each section can be thought about in the following way:

- What are your **G**oals?
  - Refer to your SMART goals for each portfolio activity: have you achieved them all or how have they changed?

- What **S**ituation are you facing?
  - What is the issue(s) that you are currently struggling with: what do you know and not know about it?

- What is your **T**hinking currently?
  - Are you making any assumptions that could be negatively affecting your career? What might others think?

- What **A**ctions are you considering?
  - What steps will you follow and do you have a timeline for these steps? What potential obstacles could arise?

- What **R**esults do you expect?
  - Do you think that the results you expect are realistic? Do you have a back-up plan if things don't work out? What potential impact could the results have on your career?

The G-Star model can be used in conjunction with Step 5 – where do you want to be? It can help you work through problems you are facing and find ways to overcome them so you can be exactly where you want to be in your career.

Again, sticking with the 'lecturing medical students' portfolio activity:

- Starting with the *Situation* – perhaps you are having issues with the pay for the sessions?

- What do you *Think* about the situation:
  - What do you know to be factually correct and what are you assuming?
  - You know the pay you are receiving, but is the rate too low? Why do you think this? What have you based your conclusion on?
  - How could you find out the average rate of pay for the session?
  - What would resolving this issue look like to you?

- What are your next steps (*Actions*) and in what order will you take them?
  - Perhaps you decide to speak to your line manager asking about the pay.
  - Perhaps you speak to a colleague who does the same job as you.
  - You might start by looking online at job adverts for similar positions.

- What could be the outcome(s) (*Results*) of the possible actions you take?
  - Could you negotiate a higher rate of pay?
  - Could there be any negative repercussions, such as affecting the professional relationship between you and your colleagues / line manager? Could this ultimately cause you to leave the job?
  - What impact could this have on your career? Could this affect you if you needed to ask for a reference for a job in the future?

5.3 Diversifying as a more experienced GP

Evaluating your career is a great opportunity to decide if you are in fact maximising your potential and doing what you truly want to be doing in your career. This is especially important if you are a more experienced GP, but you have to be completely honest with yourself. Asking yourself the following questions may help you diversify your current career options.

Do you know your worth?

Whatever stage you are at in your career, you will have gained a wealth of experience and knowledge about both clinical and non-clinical aspects to working as a GP. Add in transferable skills and your life experience to this and it is likely that you will see you are a very valuable asset both within and outside of medicine. Start by recognising that you are worth more than you may even know.

> During my FY3 year I was reminded of the surprise and excitement on people's faces when I told them I was a doctor. When I attended non-medical events and awards ceremonies, I was reminded of the respect that the public still has for doctors, even at times when it did not seem this way. I often felt much more successful and proud of myself and my career journey when I was not among medics. It seems ironic, but this was always my experience. Within the NHS I felt undervalued and unappreciated at times by both staff and patients.

If you are struggling to see how valuable you actually are, perhaps it is time to take a step away from medicine, even if only for a short holiday, and appreciate you and just how far you have come.

Do you take calculated risks?

Throughout life we sometimes have to be cautious about the decisions we make, especially if we have families to support and mortgages to pay. Having said this, it is important to be able to 'step outside the box' or out of your 'comfort zone' because this can be where the real growth occurs. What have you always wanted to do but never done? Why did you not do it? You might want to consider taking smaller steps first and try something out before committing fully. Ask yourself what would happen if you were to fail; would it affect your pride or your finances and, if so, by how much? How would this impact any future decisions you would make? Try to stay open-minded and think about the possibilities if that 'risk' were to pay off.

Have you tried and tested your hypothesis?

Leading on from the point above, sometimes we have ideas about what could work but never try them out. The only way you will know if that idea will work is to actually make it a reality. You do not have to start with a big step, it could be something small initially. You can also ask for advice and feedback from colleagues, family and friends, or even those on your social media accounts (setting up polls, for instance). Evaluating all this feedback can help guide your thought processes and decision-making.

Chapter summary

- Evaluating your career is important so you know what works, what does not and how you can constantly improve on your journey to career success.
- Accurately evaluating your career, for example by using the tools and models highlighted, will help you thoroughly discern areas that may be overlooked.
- The five-step process can be used to critically evaluate your portfolio career. Ask yourself: Where are you now? What has worked well? What has not worked so well? What can you change? Where do you want to be?
- A SWOT analysis or the G-Star model can be used in conjunction with the five-step process in the regular evaluation of your career.
- It might seem harder to make changes as a more experienced GP but it is still possible. Diversifying your career does not necessarily mean making massive changes quickly. Instead, think about taking smaller, more calculated risks that will lead you to your desired career destination.
- Finally, it helps to adopt a positive and open-minded attitude (everything we covered in *Chapter 3*!).

Chapter 6:
What is possible – learning from current portfolio GPs

This chapter will open up to you the endless opportunities available as a portfolio GP.

Through a combination of first-hand accounts and interviews you will learn why and how these incredible GPs created their portfolio careers. There are discussions around frustrations with medicine during the early part of their careers, what they are doing to improve the clinical and wider environments they work in, the importance of discovering and following their passions and seizing opportunities. A portfolio career requires time, patience, continuous evaluation of yourself and where you are in your career, as well as upskilling, being proactive and organised, and managing time effectively. There is of course much more, so read on to uncover their invaluable advice and life lessons.

When reading the stories of current portfolio GPs (and the interviews in the second part of the chapter), it is important to note that the doctors wrote about what they were doing at the time of writing; such is the nature of portfolio careers that they may now be doing different things!

6.1 Dr Safiya Virji
Medical education and leadership

Safiya Virji, MBBS BSc DFSRH MRCGP MA (Med Ed)

- Portfolio GP with a special interest in Education and Leadership
- Senior Clinical Lecturer and Deputy Head of Year 3 at Queen Mary University of London's Medical School
- Training Programme Director for GP trainees for Health Education England
- NHS GP appraiser
- Educational Supervisor for GPs in difficulty

How it all began

My most vivid memory from childhood is watching a scene on television of a female British doctor walking in a desert somewhere in Africa, being greeted by young children in ragged clothes, who took her hand and led her to a small hut to see a vulnerable family member needing medical assistance. I remember thinking, "That's the goal. That's what I want to do with my life."

Over time, my thoughts went beyond this to include: "I want to be a mother. Would my children come with me to Africa? If so, how would I look after them? If they came, how would they be educated? But if they stayed at home, when would I see them?"

As the years went on it was that scene on the TV which motivated me to work hard and overcome any obstacles which stood in my way. At medical school I soon became aware that medical pathology alone didn't excite me. It felt more like a means to an end. Treating patients in and of itself seemed like it might not be enough to satisfy me.

I noticed I was very good at organising myself and very much enjoyed identifying the difference between people's personalities and how they operated best. Having recognised a key interest area, I completed an intercalated BSc in Healthcare Management whilst at medical school, in order to see how medicine, leadership and organisational management could be combined in useful ways.

I knew that a career in general practice was the only option for me in terms of satisfying my desire to be exposed to a variety of clinical cases. I was hopeful that being a GP would help maintain my concentration and interest levels, which had wavered during my degree. I enjoyed building a rapport with patients on a grass roots level, and I knew general practice provided opportunities for a portfolio career, as well as having a reasonable enough working pattern to be there for my family.

I met my non-medic husband as I embarked on my journey as a GP trainee and through living in different towns and making new friends with people outside of the profession, I noticed that people consistently commented on my engaging, humorous and articulate nature. I often wonder whether it is my chosen profession that has brought out innate qualities or I have adopted these characteristics in response to being a medic.

Medical education

After having two children during my general practice training period, I was imminently due to qualify when my supervisor at work left a job advert on my desk for the role of Future GP Education Lead. It was an opportunity to combine general practice with education and leadership and included time to study for a Masters degree in medical education, with a day a week teaching healthcare professionals. I decided to apply.

As part of the interview, we were asked to deliver a presentation of our choice. I could see that a fellow interviewee, fully suited and booted, had prepared a PowerPoint presentation on the latest treatment guidelines for atrial fibrillation. I remember feeling I could have done with listening in on that myself.

My presentation was on potty training.

The professor of education on the interview panel spent most of my presentation snorting with laughter. It was at times like this that I knew I was different from most of the people I had trained with. Later that same day I received a phone call offering me the job.

Completing a Masters with two young children, working at a GP practice and delivering lectures was challenging, but the adrenaline was always pumping. At the time this role came to an end, I was expecting my third child. It was an opportunity to reflect on where I wanted to go in the future.

Tips for completing a Masters whilst working:

- Allocate a set time during the working week when you are most likely to be alert enough to read and absorb recommended research papers.

- Highlight quotes and sentences that interest you in everything you come across, so you can find them easily and reference them when completing future assignments.
- Try to base assignments on topics that resonate with you or are connected with / relate to what you are already doing at work, to make them more meaningful and easier to write.
- When writing assignments, start by identifying subheadings and then insert key points or bullet points under each subheading; splitting it into bite-sized chunks makes it seem less overwhelming.
- Know that whilst there are periods of high stress and pressure, these are temporary and not reflective of the entire duration of the course.

Leadership roles in education, NHS management and beyond

During my third pregnancy, I decided to use my management and educational background to apply for a part-time position as a training programme director. This proved to be an excellent opportunity to work with postgraduate doctors and help them overcome their barriers to qualify as competent and confident GPs.

On returning to work after having my third child I decided to supplement this role and reignite the management flame by applying for a position in NHS management (Clinical Director and Governing Body Member for a CCG). I noticed that colleagues enjoyed the difference in my thought process as an educator, and the simplicity and clarity that I brought to the table. I supplemented this with working as an out-of-hours GP so I could fit this around my children's schedules, often working after putting them to bed.

After two and a half years of this relatively stable set-up, I felt my progress had stalled and it was time to leave the CCG and complement and enhance my position as a training programme director through an alternative educational leadership position. I applied for a senior position as an undergraduate educator at a medical school. Acquiring this position was a competitive and lengthy process because senior academics there were concerned about the vast differences in how postgraduate and undergraduate medical education are delivered in the UK. It has been a steep learning curve but that's what attracts me to new roles. The prospect of growth fills me with enthusiasm and satisfaction about making the most of my career and my life.

My interest in different personalities and my commitment to supporting doctors in difficulty also led to my becoming an NHS GP appraiser. I carve time out of my life to facilitate conversations around how GPs can be the best versions of themselves, both personally and professionally. This stems from my belief in a growth mindset as a means to optimising success and wellbeing.

More recently my experience in supporting doctors in difficulty led to my becoming an educational supervisor for qualified GPs who have conditions on practice. I am invested in improving the GP workforce dilemma and have always been willing to tackle recruitment and retention of GPs through whatever means possible. Supporting GPs to recover from significant events at work and practise safely is another way to stabilise the GP workforce.

There were points during my career where I was worn out from my contributions to the NHS. I often recalled how this wasn't even what inspired me to do medicine! What happened to the scene on television?!

Tips for avoiding burnout

- Take time out regularly to assess your work–life balance and whether either of these is being neglected.
- Be realistic and create opportunities that will fit in with your life.
- Consider flexible working to enable you to do the things that are most important to you.

In 2016 I was offered the opportunity to support a UK-based charity operating in the Middle East providing voluntary medical care to orphans and the vulnerable. My children were very young and I wondered if this was the right time to take on such a commitment. I decided to forge ahead. In the years since, I have become the clinic lead for the charity, running medical camps up to three times a year offering free medical care to those that need it most in regions torn apart by war. It is by far the most satisfying, heart-warming, and the most humbling part of my life and my career. And as for the kids… they often travel with me, and it has shaped them to be compassionate and generous humans, which is more important to me than anything else. In terms of their education I've realised that there are no better lifelong learning lessons than those which come from immersing yourself in charity work. Their schools have always been supportive of my work and are understanding if the children have had to miss a few days of school due to travel.

Tips for working / volunteering in the charity sector

- Voluntary work abroad is great for learning about different cultures and behaviours. Often there's a lot to learn from the people you meet that enhances your life in varying ways at home in the UK.
- Taking regular breaks from NHS work can be great for wellbeing and work–life balance, and experiencing alternative patient behaviours and demands can be energising.
- Portfolio careers allow for additional flexibility, and taking time off is often easier due to the variable contract styles of non-clinical work.

Pros and cons to a portfolio career and how to overcome any challenges

Pros:

- Portfolio careers can act as a means to maintaining wellbeing, as you keep your mind active through the pursuit of side interests outside of your core qualifications.
- It can provide a flexible way of working as it's widely expected that portfolio meetings and specialist services would work around core clinical or personal commitments.
- Portfolio interests can develop as you evolve – unlike your core qualification, you can pursue certain specialist areas as much as you want or change and start new ones. It allows for creativity and freedom within the work context.

Cons:

- Having more than one job can require significant organisation in terms of timetabling. However, this is usually a career choice and therefore activities would be chosen by you!
- Annual leave may need to be pursued through more than one establishment if you want a block of time off; however, this has luckily never been a problem for me personally!
- It can be tiring. Portfolio careers can sometimes require courses or additional preparation which can be tiring if you are doing this after a full day of work. Always keeping the bigger picture at the forefront of your mind can help keep up the motivation to get through those difficult evenings.

In summary, as a GP with a successful portfolio career, my advice to anyone looking to pursue a similar career path is that it is important to reflect regularly on where your interest lies. Portfolio careers tend to work best when you offset the extra organisational requirements with waking up every day excited about what the day holds. When you feel comfortable with your set-up, this is the time to think about how you could increase your skill set to open up other opportunities for growth. The more experience and exposure you have to different things, the more interesting and rare opportunities you will find yourself suitable to undertake. When something is not fun any more or it's not what you thought it would be, move on! There are so many opportunities that can be excellent stepping stones towards your dream portfolio career!

This is my story, it's time to create yours!

6.2 Dr Aman Amir
GP partner, university lecturer, magistrate and author

Aman Amir, MBChB, FRCGP, DRFSRH, SFHEA, JP

- GP partner
- University lecturer
- Magistrate
- Author

How it all began

I was 8 years old when I won a local painting competition. This created quite a stir and before I knew it, I was on local radio and television. I'll never forget the question, *"So do you think you'll become a famous painter when you grow up?"*.

I'll also never forget my reply, *"No I'm going to be a doctor when I grow up."*

But no one had asked what kind of doctor I wanted to be. I had such a wide range of interests growing up and even at university. It always felt like I had to give something up in order to proceed further into my medical career. We would all agree that a degree of sacrifice is needed when trying to achieve great things.

Having thoroughly enjoyed medical school and all it had to offer, I was thrust into being a junior doctor back in 2002. With no formal careers advice to lean on, I was lucky to have found great mentors and, under close guidance from them, I embarked on a surgical career.

Those years spent in hospital medicine were certainly not a waste of time. I am so grateful to have been exposed to various hospitals and departments and medical experiences, and most of all I've gained great insight into patient journeys and had the opportunity to care for people with a wide range of illnesses. All of which has helped me to perform as an empathetic and holistic GP in the community.

The constant stream of on-calls, nightshifts and social sacrifices was beginning to take a heavy toll on me and my family life and eventually I gave in to my need for balance. Finally, I felt ready to become who I wanted to be when I made my decision as a child to be a doctor. A lot had happened in my life between the age of 8 and qualifying as a doctor, not least of all my father being diagnosed with cancer and dying even before I set foot in medical school.

Soon after gaining my MRCGP, I was offered some teaching work for the university. Having spent so many years in hospital medicine where I enjoyed supporting medical students, it became obvious to me that this was something I would enjoy more in future and possibly need to formalise as a role. It's now been over a decade that I've been a university lecturer delivering various sessions and sitting on interview panels and examining for the medical school. This role facilitated my completion of Senior Fellowship from the Higher Education Academy (SFHEA).

Senior Fellowship of the Higher Education Academy (SFHEA)

This is awarded to professionals who demonstrate they meet certain criteria of high standards for teaching and supporting learning in higher education (see www.advance-he.ac.uk/fellowship/senior-fellowship).

A sustained record of effectiveness in teaching and learning, organisation and leadership, along with management with regard to teaching and learning provision, has to be demonstrated. This is awarded to experienced staff able to demonstrate the impact and influence that their methods have had on the learning community.

Proficiency must be demonstrated in some key areas:

- Knowledge – core knowledge and teaching theory
- Professional values
- Engagement
- Research activity
- Continuous professional development.

A written reflective account of practice including two case studies, along with a supporting statement from two referees, is submitted for assessment by the panel.

The Higher Education Academy awards in seniority are as follow:

- Associate Fellow
- Fellow
- Senior Fellow
- Principal Fellow.

During my GP training I undertook further studies in sexual health, gaining my Diploma from the Faculty of Sexual and Reproductive Health (DFSRH).

Diploma from the Faculty of Sexual and Reproductive Health (DFSRH)

Be sure to make sure you fulfil the entry requirements (see www. fsrh.org/education-and-training/diploma):

- Be registered with a UK or Irish medical professional body and have a licence to practise
- Be able to administer an intramuscular injection
- Be able to administer a subcutaneous injection
- Be able to perform a speculum examination
- Be up to date with resuscitation and anaphylaxis training in line with UK guidelines
- Be able to commit to the learning programme and accept the learning charter.

The course covers topics such as anatomy and physiology, risk assessment and history-taking, contraceptive choices, emergency contraception, planning for pregnancy and how to manage side-effects of contraception.

There is an independent learning portfolio that you need to work through in addition to successfully passing:

- an online theory assessment
- a summative clinical assessment
- a half-day assessment.

So, once you have made sure you are eligible, you need to find a faculty that is registered in training and then apply for the Diploma. You will need to complete the training within 2 years of starting the programme.

Following evaluation, you will receive the DFSRH and can then look for further training into specific areas of interest within sexual health.

Finally, you will need to recertify every 5 years to maintain the accreditation.

At no stage did I set out to become a 'portfolio GP'. This was a term an appraiser once used to describe my working week. I divided my time between clinical sessions at the practice and time during the week teaching at the university, along with other outside interests such as writing and court. Not to mention my hobbies!

I joined the Magistrates' Bench some years ago, following my call to civic duty, which I find extremely rewarding, along with my interest in writing fiction. Both these endeavours have helped me grow as an individual and indeed as a GP. It wouldn't be possible to pursue either of these activities if I had a rigid working week like I did when I worked in the hospitals.

Magistrate (Justice of the Peace)

If you have a strong sense of civic duty and want to give back, and are aged between 18 and 74, this might be something of interest to you (see www.gov.uk/become-magistrate/can-you-be-a-magistrate).

Personal qualities you should have:

- Awareness of social issues
- Maturity and understanding of people
- A sense of fairness and equality
- Reliability and commitment to community
- Ability to think logically and weigh up arguments
- Effective communicator
- Good character (previous convictions can affect the application).

You should spend some time in court observing, because several sittings are required prior to applying. Candidates will be called for an interview where the panel will go through the application and ask questions relating to interests and motivation for becoming a magistrate. If successful, the next stage will be an assessment day. This involves some time to analyse various scenarios in a quiet room alone. This is followed by questions relating to the scenarios by a panel. Here the candidate is expected to explain the rationale and methodology regarding the outcomes of those scenarios. The candidate's problem-solving skills are being assessed more deeply here.

Once this stage is passed, official training is offered. There are several courses and training days covering a variety of cases and guidelines. Each new magistrate is also allocated a mentor who supports and works with the magistrate towards appraisals and completion of various courses and continuous professional development.

Once completed, the magistrate is part of the judiciary and can keep up to date with various developments and pursue further training in areas of interest.

Author

If you enjoy reading and escapism or words, then maybe writing fiction might be a great hobby to pursue. Here are some tips for how you might get started:

- Attending local and national workshops
- Writing festivals can be very inspiring and helpful for beginners
- A course in writing can help or you could pursue higher education in English language
- Joining a writing or peer group can be very helpful and provide support as well.

If you really enjoying writing and want to progress further, it might be an idea to get a literary agent who can help with getting works published, or alternatively one can self-publish. Writing non-fiction might be the usual route because one can concentrate on an area of expertise and write with a certain group in mind for whom the work is targeted. Either way, writing requires some of these skills and qualities:

- Passion and desire
- Dedication and discipline
- Organisation and focus.

As with most things, speaking to people in that field and making a network of supportive allies always helps you on your journey.

During the pandemic it became increasingly evident how difficult things have become in primary care from an organisation and service provision point of view, and just how important it is to maintain a healthy work–life balance doing what you enjoy and being appropriately rewarded.

Thanks to the flexibility I created in my working week I was able to also care for my mother during her terminal illness. Sadly, she passed away in June 2022 following treatments for cancer. We doctors are humans as well and we have families and lives that also need our time and attention.

My working week looks like this:

- Mondays and Fridays – teaching
- Tuesdays and Thursdays – clinical work
- Wednesdays – court day
- Weekends – some clinical / administrative work.

Advice about working as a portfolio GP

Working hard to forge a career in medicine is very difficult and takes many years to achieve, and after such a mountain has been climbed, one needs to be able to find the strength to prosper and continue in such a competitive and stressful environment.

Increasingly therefore, GPs have looked to create a portfolio of work that captures their imagination and drives their motivation, and this has become a sought-after approach for budding GPs.

My advice is that one should really enjoy what one is pursuing, whatever the career path. It is fair to say the harder we work, the more pleasure we also get (in most cases). So, the main thing is to discover what we like and enjoy and feel our investment of time and energy would be worth it.

Use time at medical school to speak with clinical supervisors and find good mentors. Try to get the most out of attachments – this might be the most exposure you get in that field before choosing your path.

Get your head around the exams and especially the postgraduate requirements for the specialty and, if you have a special interest, explore what needs to be done to get the relevant accreditations. This includes costs and the time that needs to be invested in this pursuit. Being organised and devoted, with some guidance along the way, will help the majority with their pursuits.

Look at your week and how you would like to spend it. Some may want to split their clinical work into general practice and specialist interest, and others turn to creativity to help balance out and add to their personal fulfilment. However your working is planned or whatever it looks like, you need to be able to sustain it and keep interested in it in order to give the best to your patients and colleagues.

Good luck!

6.3 Dr Daniel Grace
Expedition medicine

Daniel Grace, MBBS, BSc (Hons), Dip EWM, DTMH, MRCGP (2017), MFTM, RCPS (Glas), FRGS

- Locum GP
- Travel health physician
- Medical educator
- GP appraiser
- Event and expedition doctor
- Volunteer as the medical director for 'The Virtual Doctors', a leading telemedicine charity, and Medserve Wales, a pre-hospital care organisation based in South Wales

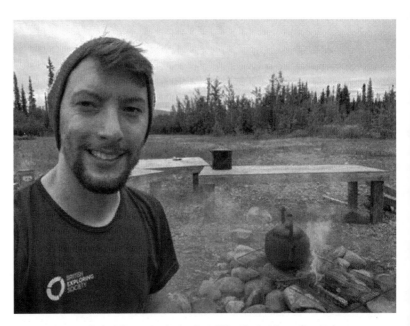

Supporting youth development through trekking in the Canadian Yukon.

How it all began

If I rewind to the penultimate few months of my GP ST3 year, I could tell that I was not going to suit a 'normal' GP job, and that the standard model of partnership or salaried general practice was not for me. In fact, I toyed with the idea of leaving medicine at this point, but I wasn't really sure what I could do instead that would offer me the same level of flexibility and pay. As I write this, I am pleased that I chose to persevere with general practice, albeit playing to my own rules. Whilst my Vocational Training Scheme (VTS) contemporaries started their salaried or partnership jobs, I decided a few weeks hiking in the Julian Alps in Slovenia was the perfect way to celebrate becoming a GP.

Expedition medicine

A few weeks prior to this I had attended an expedition and wilderness medicine course run by World Extreme Medicine, using my study budget which I had saved up by refusing to book onto any AKT or CSA revision courses. I remember I had picked up a brochure for one of these courses at a careers fair when I was an F2, and I had always thought it sounded interesting. As I suspected, it was a fascinating week of talks, practical sessions and scenario-based teaching, which culminated in a simulated search and rescue exercise. I was hooked; however, the most important thing for me at this point in my career was not necessarily the medicine or the course content, but the fact that I had discovered a community of like-minded medics who wanted to develop alternative careers that were outside of the traditional confines of what we had been sold at medical school.

From here I set about working out how to develop my interest in expedition medicine, whilst doing ad hoc locum general practice work to pay the bills. I decided to study for the International Diploma in Expedition and Wilderness Medicine, run by the Royal College of Physicians and Surgeons in Glasgow.

This diploma was a blended mixture of remote learning and residential placements, which made it ideal to complete whilst I continued to pick up locum work. Some particular highlights included winter skills training at Glenmore Lodge in Scotland, and spending time out in the mountains and deserts of Morocco, where we were put through our paces managing simulated casualties. Since then I have provided medical support for multiple endurance events and treks in a wide range of environments, including the tea plantations of Kenya, the deserts of Jordan and the wilderness of the Canadian Yukon. I have also worked in the South Pacific to support the filming of a major US TV series. Closer to home I have worked on various multi-day ultramarathons and the Ride Across Britain Land's End to John o' Groats cycling event. These events are always great fun, and you meet so many inspiring characters – both staff and participants alike.

These aforementioned jobs have been a mixture of voluntary and paid work, with some trips covering expenses and therefore being cost neutral. Unfortunately, it is unlikely that expedition medicine will replace general practice when it comes to paying bills and mortgages; however, it is an excellent way to travel and feel refreshed and inspired. It also gives you many transferable skills to use when back working in the NHS. Obviously, this type of work dried up overnight during the height of the Covid pandemic, but the travel industry appears to have bounced back, and there is still substantial demand for expedition medics at the time of writing. As GPs, with our generalist backgrounds, we are ideally placed to manage the wide range of problems which may occur on an expedition. That being said, it is important to ensure that you have appropriate emergency medicine and pre-hospital training to deal with any accidents or injuries that may arise in an austere environment, and completing a pre-hospital trauma life support course should be considered as a minimum requirement.

To get involved:

- Complete a practical expedition medicine course or diploma. The following list is by no means exhaustive but a good place to start:
  - World Extreme Medicine: www.worldextrememedicine.com
  - Unique Expeditions: www.uniqueexpeditions.co.uk
  - Royal College of Physicians and Surgeons of Glasgow: rcpsg. ac.uk/travel-medicine/qualifications-in-travel-medicine/ rcpsg-international-postgraduate-diploma-in-expedition-and-wilderness-medicine
  - Mountain Medicine Diploma: www.uclan.ac.uk/postgraduate/ courses/mountain-medicine-msc
  - Remote Area Risk International: www.r2rinternational.com
  - Endeavour Medical: endeavourmedical.co.uk

- Consider completing a pre-hospital trauma life support (PHTLS) course, which is recognised around the world as the leading continuing education programme for pre-hospital emergency trauma.
- Get used to working outside your comfort zone.
- Start working on UK-based events. There are lots of different organisations looking for medics with a range of experiences. A good way to start is by contacting local event organisers.
- Graduate to working on low-risk overseas expeditions.

If expedition and wilderness medicine is something you want to find out more about, please have a look at my website www. thewildernessmedic.com where I write about my experiences in more detail. Another useful website which is well worth checking out is www.theadventuremedic.com where you will find blogs, articles, course reviews and more.

Medical education

Since delving into the world of expedition medicine, I have started teaching on various expedition medicine courses, which has been a great way to remain up-to-date and active in the wilderness medicine community. This is usually face-to-face teaching, similar to the courses that I did myself. However, I have also written content for the new online diploma and MSc programme in Expedition and Wilderness Medicine run by the University of South Wales, and it was great to be able to shape and develop a completely new course. It has also been really valuable to hone my teaching skills, and I have been able to transfer these across to some primary care roles through teaching medical students at King's College London and Swansea Medical School as part of their undergraduate general practice curriculum. Many of these job opportunities have arisen from sending lots of emails and joining lots of Zoom calls. Not every exciting opportunity will be what it says on the tin and unfortunately you have to be prepared to put in the legwork and accept that you may go down several dead ends before you reach your destination. That does not mean that the skills you have gained on the journey are redundant, and I am often pleasantly surprised how various threads of my career have subsequently joined up.

One of these connected themes has been clinical simulation, which nicely links together my roles in general practice, expedition medicine and pre-hospital medicine. As I am at different stages in each of these fields, I am able to experience simulation both as a facilitator and a participant, which is hugely valuable. In 2019 several GP colleagues and I in the southeast of England decided to create a pilot programme that aimed to bring simulation into the domain of primary care. We felt that simulation thus far had been predominantly reserved for secondary care and hospital trainees, but also that it didn't have to be this way, and the benefits of simulation were equally relevant in the community setting.

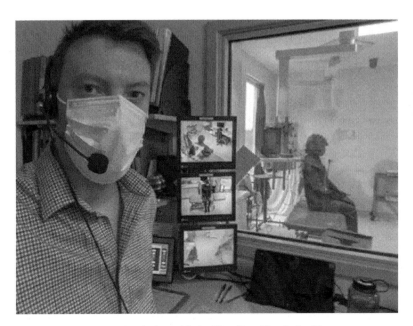

Running primary care simulation with the West Kent Simulation Team.

One of the many issues affecting general practice at the time of writing, surrounds the interface between primary care and the ambulance service, with increasing demands being placed on primary care teams, when managing acutely unwell patients. As a result of numerous factors, GPs are seeing a greater number of later presentations and acutely unwell patients. On top of this, we are having to manage these unwell patients in the community for longer, and as a "place of safety" ambulance resources are often diverted to other calls. This pilot scheme was therefore well received by experienced GPs, practice nurses, HCAs and trainees alike, and we received excellent feedback, being nominated for the Patient Safety Awards in 2021. Now that I have moved to the other side of the UK, I am in the process of creating a similar programme in South Wales. I believe that there is substantial value in being able to practise managing an emergency in a safe protected learning environment, and that the opportunity to work through and discuss this with peers can really generate positive change.

To get involved:

- Think laterally: if you have an interest in education, see if you can teach people about what you already know
- It is possible to develop an interest without a formal qualification; however, a diploma or similar may be beneficial if you hope to get involved with academia or lecturing.

Medserve Wales and pre-hospital care

One of the challenges with developing a portfolio career is ensuring that you remain up to date with the various competencies required for each role you carry out. For me it was important to supplement my general practice and expedition medicine roles with some UK-based pre-hospital care experience. This was something that I had been looking to do for several years and in 2021 I was lucky enough to join the Medserve Wales team as a trainee. Medserve is a branch of the British Association of Immediate Care (BASICS) based in South Wales and is made up of a multidisciplinary team of volunteer doctors, nurses and paramedics who provide enhanced care to support the Welsh Ambulance Service. As one of only two GPs in the team, I am really pleased to be involved, and whilst I am at the start of my formal pre-hospital career, my eventual aim is to pass the Diploma in Immediate Care set by the Faculty of Pre-hospital Care, based at the Royal College of Surgeons Edinburgh. Until then, in my spare time I get to receive expert training from inspiring pre-hospital practitioners, participate in multi-agency simulation training, and head out on shift in DR-01, our response car, to support the ambulance service. As mentioned, participating in simulation sessions, whilst sometimes nerve-wracking, is a great way to learn and stress-test your own competencies in a safe environment.

To get involved:

- Try to get some pre-hospital experience and qualifications, such as the PHTLS, as discussed above
- Identify your local British Association for Immediate Care (BASICS) scheme, Search and Rescue team or Mountain Rescue team:
  - www.basics.org.uk
  - www.lowlandrescue.org
  - www.mountain.rescue.org.uk
- Express your interest and ask questions – you might be surprised where you end up!

The Virtual Doctors

The final role that I will share with you is my volunteer position as the medical director for the Virtual Doctors. The Virtual Doctors is a UK-based charity that uses a bespoke smartphone app to connect isolated health centres in rural Zambia with volunteer doctors, based predominantly in the UK. These doctors offer advice to diagnose conditions and treat patients, which assists and empowers rural health workers and their communities, whilst reducing the number of hospital referrals that would incur long, arduous journeys and unmanageable expense. I first joined as a volunteer in 2018, a year or so after gaining my CCT, and found it really rewarding and interesting to answer cases. Naturally when the charity asked for expressions of interest to join the medical team, I applied and further on down the road I took on the role of medical director. This is a stimulating and varied role that has given me a real insight into the complexities of running a charity. My role involves meetings with potential technological or healthcare partners, writing grants and policies, giving talks, recruiting and vetting volunteers and of course answering cases. This role has also allowed me to appreciate the challenges of healthcare delivery on a global scale and has illustrated the importance of ensuring equitable healthcare. The Covid-19 pandemic revealed that telemedical technology has huge potential in healthcare; however, we must be careful to ensure that this also benefits patients in low-resource settings. This is something that the Virtual Doctors can be at the forefront of, so it is a very exciting time for the charity! We are always keen to invite new volunteer doctors to join our team, especially if you have experience of working in sub-Saharan Africa or similar low-resource settings; please visit virtualdoctors.org for more information or to get in touch.

I hope this has given a flavour of some of the potential roles you can incorporate into a portfolio career. Whilst general practice is at the root, and indeed it is necessary to remain financially secure, it has also opened many doors to other areas that I had not even considered were possible when I obtained my CCT. I won't lie and say it didn't take hard work and persistence, but I think medicine can open many doors if you knock on the right ones. Even if you don't find the right one to start with, walking through the doorway can often reveal the greatest opportunities.

6.4 Dr Ellen Welch
Remote working, medical journalism and cruise ship doctor

Ellen Welch, MBChB, BA (Hons), MRCEM, MRCGP (2013), DTMH, DFSRH

- GP working from home doing a combination of e-consults, OOH telephone triage and call reviews for a local practice and a national NHS OOH provider
- Co-chair of the Doctors' Association UK
- Medical journalist
- Cruise ship doctor
- Ski field medic in New Zealand
- Expedition doctor
- Glastonbury Festival Medic

How it all began

Being 'portfolio' was never in my game plan, but I knew from very early on in my career that I wanted to use medicine to travel. I qualified in 2004 from Liverpool Medical School, taking an extra year as a student to intercalate in medical journalism in London. After a year of house jobs back in Liverpool, I moved to New Zealand, spending a happy year as a 'medical reliever'. This is a uniquely New Zealand position, similar to being a locum, but being a salaried employee, on hand to cover junior doctor rota gaps – which allowed me to get a taste of a broad range of specialities. The ethos in New Zealand was very refreshing compared to the culture of the NHS. I felt very much part of the team, despite rotating quite frequently. Consultants socialised with their teams. We had a bar in the doctors' mess (hell, we had a doctors' mess, which is more than the UK can boast these days) and pizza and beers after work on a Friday were standard. Food was free each day. Time out of training was actively encouraged and the work–life balance worked.

I returned to the UK to undertake the Diploma in Tropical Medicine back in Liverpool for 3 months, and then took up a 6-month stand-alone position, to gain more experience, as an SHO in Emergency Medicine in Yorkshire. *Modernising Medical Careers* was being implemented (a change in the organisation of training pathways) around this time, causing chaos for a 'lost tribe' of SHOs, and I got caught up in the whole scramble for training positions, and spent a further 2 years training in emergency medicine in Leeds. I got some emergency medicine exams under my belt (MCEM), then got itchy feet again. I had been looking into working on cruise ships for about a year, and after the intensity of exams and ED shift work, I was elated to line up a position on a ship in the Caribbean during the UK winter.

Work as a cruise ship doctor

My first contract was a full 6 months on board sailing around the Caribbean. I had lined up a winter role in New Zealand following this contract, spending a ski season in Queenstown as a ski field medic (best job ever…). I then bounced from cruise ships to UK locums for a few years (with some festival medical work thrown in there), before deciding to return to the UK to undertake GP training. As a cruise ship doctor I was looking after the hard-working crew members as well as the passengers – I was their GP, and I realised I valued this continuity of care. In many countries, doctors are GPs as soon as they come out of medical school, so I had a few bemused colleagues on board when I told them I was returning home to train to be a GP.

As a cruise ship doctor, you do really need to be ready to deal with anything. Ships are floating cities, and the biggest in the world (currently the *Symphony of the Seas*) has a capacity of nearly 9000 passengers and crew.

The size of medical teams vary – the standard team is made up of two doctors, three nurses and a medical secretary, with bigger ships employing up to three doctors. I've also worked on smaller vessels as a solo doctor. This does mean that you are constantly on call. You do devise your own rota and have downtime, but there is always the possibility of an emergency. Salary depends on length of service but ranges from £8k to 14k per month on board (vacations are unpaid); you also obviously get a room, a one-minute commute to work and access to the all-you-can-eat buffets, meaning there are opportunities to save.

Clinics run daily for three hours in the morning (8am–11am) and three hours in the afternoon (4pm–7pm). Some days clinics will be packed full, with a mix of minor complaints and often fairly significant medical problems. Other days may be quieter when the ship is docked and everyone wants to explore. The role is unique within medicine and you may be managing a crew member's hypertension one moment, and then get summoned by an emergency 'alpha call' to a trauma on the pool deck, or a cardiac arrest in a guest cabin. Coughs and colds sit alongside patients needing respiratory support. Accidents and their investigation are bread and butter, and the ability to suture and cast fractures is essential.

The onboard medical facility is equipped with an X-ray machine, blood test equipment and a well-stocked pharmacy, alongside both ward and intensive care unit (ICU) facilities set up to manage critically ill patients for several days – which is a must when the ship crosses the Atlantic – a journey that takes five days and is too far from land to coordinate a heli-evac (an evacuation from the ship via helicopter). It is possible to carry out blood transfusions at sea – reserved for only the most critical cases, when care on land is too far away – and I was involved in several of these cases. Coordinating the logistics of this is one of the most rewarding aspects of the job, seeing the whole of the ship pull together – guests and crew helping out a fellow traveller. When a passenger needs further care on land, it's a team effort, working alongside the navigational bridge, security, guest services (to name but a few) to ensure disembarkation takes place safely and smoothly, whether that's by speeding the ship up to reach land faster, or slowing it down to allow a helicopter to hover above and winch a patient to safety.

Public health is a huge part of the job (even more so since the pandemic) and the medical team must be prepared to manage any outbreaks of disease, and ensure the ship maintains standards for health inspections. Crew vaccination programmes are coordinated by the medical team, alongside crew wellness programmes and teaching crew basic life support. Being senior doctor also involves managing the medical team, and liaising with all the other departments on board, attending management meetings, crew drills and showing your face on the stage in front of guests during formal nights.

Working all over the world brings its own challenges, but after some time, you find yourself becoming familiar with the logistics in different ports of call, and befriending port agents to help organise shoreside care for passengers unable to continue with their cruise.

Requirements to work as a cruise ship doctor:

- GMC registration and at least three years of postgraduate work with clinical experience in emergency medicine, acute care or ICU. There is flexibility here and you can discuss your experience on an individual basis.
- Hold accredited certificates in Advanced Life Support (ALS) or the American Advanced Cardiac Life Support (ACLS), Advanced

Paediatric Life Support (APLS) or Paediatric Life Support (https://cpr.heart.org/en/courses/pals-course-options), or Advanced Trauma Life Support (ATLS).

- A valid passport and a United States C1/D visa (companies will assist you to obtain this).
- Competency in advanced airway management (intubation / conscious sedation); the ability to reduce common fractures / dislocations and suture wounds; management of cardiac events and the ability to lead a cardiac arrest team.

My ten years at sea was intermingled with NHS work to ensure I was able to revalidate and, in 2010, inspired by my work as a family doctor onboard, I spent three years training to be a GP in Cumbria (using my annual leave to do short stints at sea to keep up my skills). I rotated through useful hospital specialities including obstetrics and gynaecology, psychiatry and ENT (working for a consultant who I first met at sea when their relative was admitted to our medical facility!). After completing my training and gaining my Certificate of Completion of Training (CCT), I moved to take up a salaried position in West London. I worked eight sessions and did OOH work alongside. I also started doing intermittent repatriation work – escorting patients who had fallen ill overseas back to the UK.

After a relationship breakdown, I returned once again to sea full-time in 2015, this time as a senior doctor, and did several back-to-back contracts on the same ship. Contracts were four months on, three months off, so I returned to GP work in London in the breaks, travelled, continued my repatriation work and took opportunities as they arose – including a stint as an expedition doctor, joining a team of Canadian celebrities up Kilimanjaro, and telemedicine GP work with Dr Morton's.

I loved working at sea. It is a unique environment, and it was a privilege to live and work alongside fantastic people from all over the world. I visited every continent bar Antarctica, I learned how to scuba dive whilst on board, I wrote some books and I met my husband. During 2018, after ten years at sea, we returned to the UK to start a family.

Remote work as a GP

Immediately after returning to land, I worked as a salaried OOH doctor in Cumbria, doing mainly evenings and night shifts. In the run-up to the arrival of my first child, I signed up to do remote OOH work, mindful of the fact I would not be getting NHS maternity pay due to my travels. I tried to do a handful of shifts each week, which worked out more than maternity allowance would have provided, whilst still being able to stay at home with my babies (often working from bed, breastfeeding). I also had plans to possibly live overseas in my husband's home country, and continue the NHS work remotely, but the pandemic hit, and I've continued to work from home ever since.

Currently I work as a remote GP which includes OOH care, e-consults and telephone consultations. Alongside the remote work, I am (at the time of writing) also co-chair of the Doctors' Association UK – which I became part of during the pandemic – initially as editorial lead, with the aim to use my writing skills to campaign for doctors. This is an unpaid voluntary role, but often feels like a full-time job.

A typical working week for me is coordinated around childcare. My boys go to nursery three days a week and I do two e-consult sessions on those days. I have 24 patients per session – which is a lot, but often there is an element of triage; if a patient clearly needs to be examined, for example, I will arrange a face-to-face review, so many consults can be quick triage decisions, or a quick Med 3, whereas others are more involved. I usually schedule one of my sessions in the evening, to give me breathing space to cook and do nursery pick-ups, but often if I have time I will do these evening consults during nursery time.

Current roles:

- **Remote OOH GP** – I started this role pre-pandemic when pregnant with my first child, as it offered an opportunity to work from home and work around my baby. There are now several OOH companies set up to do this work; I work for a company which provides OOH cover and works alongside NHS 111 in several locations in the UK. The very nature of the work means the hours are typically weekends, evenings and nights, although the link with 111 means there are daytime shifts offered as a GP dealing with 111 queries. The role does also offer face-to-face and home visiting work for GPs living near base. I don't do this, but I do some Lead GP work within this role, which has involved interviewing new GPs, but at present is mainly call reviews – assessing colleagues' telephone consultations (all GPs get quarterly call reviews carried out, which are great for appraisals).

- **Locum GP** – I work remotely for a number of local practices in Cumbria, doing an average of six sessions a week. This role developed during the pandemic and I started doing e-consults with my old training practice. I took on the role while pregnant with baby number two and continued when he was born. The flexibility of the role is what has made this work for me. I have a list of 24 patients (e-consults) with no fixed timeslots and I can consult around childcare. If patients need a call then I do that; face-to-face appointments are arranged with colleagues, and many consults such as fit note requests simply require an SMS response. This role has recently expanded to other local practices, which have seen the benefits of using a remote workforce, with local knowledge, so I now work at several other practices in the area doing e-consults, telephone calls and admin. I have access to a network of other remote GPs and local study days, and benefit from having trained in the area, meaning I know colleagues in different practices which makes it easier to ask questions and approach them for help; these are all important considerations when being fairly isolated at home.

Working the way I do now is a million miles away from my previous work as a cruise ship doctor. I transitioned from being in charge of a busy ship's medical facility and all that entailed (coordinating often dramatic heli-evacs for scared patients and their families, transfusing patients at sea, dealing with cardiac arrests, psych cases and all the quirks of referring to different hospitals all over the world), to sitting in front of a computer, with my (usually sleeping) babies next to me, dealing with e-consults and telephone calls. Stressful in a different way, much more sedate, but a job that very much suits this time of my life and offers a flexibility I am grateful for.

Medical journalism

I wanted to be a journalist before I even wanted to be a doctor, and jumped at the chance to intercalate in medical journalism as a student. During this degree I started writing a lot of articles for the *Student BMJ* and *BMJ Careers*, and the writing has continued alongside my clinical work, both in mainstream media and trade press. I've written for *The Times, The Guardian, The Independent, Mail Plus, Metro, Huff Post, Pulse, GPOnline* and the *BMJ*, alongside many medical journals. I've also written several books about the NHS and an award-winning workbook to help GP Registrars pass their clinical exams.

Here are some tips to get you started in this field:

- Know your audience – don't be afraid to contact publishers directly to pitch your ideas, but before doing so prepare by checking about their style and seeing if they have any guidelines for authors. Be prepared with and have specific ideas about what you can offer.

- Start small – websites, blogs and smaller publications may be a good starting point (the Doctors' Association UK is always happy to accept blogs from doctors and medical students at press@dauk.org). As a GP Registrar I wrote for *Innovait,* the magazine for GP trainees. Websites and blogs have also taken off since I started; these are all good options for getting started in writing. The *Writers' and Artists' Yearbook* is a good source of information on publications / contacts, and often mainstream publications will be interested in first-person voices. The Medical Journalists' Association is a great source of contacts and also jobs.

- Make it relevant – when pitching to mainstream media, think about how your contribution ties into the latest news stories; if you can find a relevant news 'hook' and a fresh angle then this is helpful; these outlets are typically interested in hearing first-person voices.

- Know your worth – I think that as a group, doctors undervalue themselves. I have been paid for some of my writing, but for the vast majority of my work I haven't and I've done it for the platform the publication has given or, with many of the books, donated any royalties to charity. Medics are typically not even offered a fee for writing for some outlets, who see it as an opportunity to have a platform for their work. In contrast, most journalists wouldn't dream of putting hours of effort into an unpaid article! My tip to aspiring writers would be to throw off the medic mindset of writing for your CV or the experience, and charge the same fees as a journalist – this is work after all.

The Doctors' Association UK

The DAUK work fits in where it can. DAUK is a non-profit lobbying organisation representing UK doctors and medical students, formed on the back of the 2016 junior doctor strikes, to speak up for frontline doctors and the NHS. A lot of the DAUK team joined the organisation during the pandemic, as we watched healthcare workers risking their lives and giving their all in the fight against Covid-19. Many of us were inspired to speak up during this time, and counter a lot of the misinformation and negative narratives about Covid, vaccines and general practice. Speaking to the media isn't something doctors are trained to do, and usually actively avoid for a multitude of reasons. DAUK offers a voice to the profession, and we routinely put forward our experiences in print, on radio and TV, as a group of working GPs, consultants and junior doctors from a broad range of specialties. We have also conducted several MP briefings on the NHS. Alongside the general issues we campaign for, we also help individuals with our 'learn not blame' team – who famously helped Dr Hadiza Bawa-Garba through her gross negligence manslaughter case.

Practically, we have weekly meetings with our paid admin team to plan the week's work, events and press releases. Our committee of volunteer doctors generally meets every fortnight, but we have daily communication on our campaigns and media appearances. The fact we are a small organisation does allow us to be nimble and responsive to events, and journalists approach us almost daily for comment. Some weeks can be extremely busy sorting out campaign work, writing letters or opinion pieces, whereas other weeks can be quieter.

Summary

The NHS is not an easy place to work in the current climate. I feel very strongly that I would have burnt out a long time ago if I had pursued a more traditional career path within the NHS. For me, I'm unsure what the future holds for my career – I wouldn't rule out a return to sea one day (with appropriate re-training) and I am likely to return to face-to-face appointments once my children grow older. As a GP, there is a huge misunderstanding from the public (and non-GP NHS staff) about what the job involves, and a very negative attitude to 'part-timers' who 'lack vocation' by pursuing other interests. My advice to anyone keen to follow the portfolio route is to go for it wholeheartedly. We are fortunate enough to work in a profession that offers so many interesting avenues to explore, and which can take us around the world. As clichéd as it is to say this, we only have one life and it goes ever so quickly. We have all spent our twenties in front of textbooks and on long hospital placements to become doctors – and doing this job is a real privilege – but it can also take its toll as we all know, so we need to ensure we follow our passions.

6.5 Dr Talha Sami
Author, media contributor and content creator

Talha Sami, MBBS, iBSc, MA, MRCGP

- Locum GP
- Author and media contributor
- Content creator

How it all began

I went directly through my GCSEs and A-levels to studying at UCL and St George's, University of London, completing my F1 and F2 immediately after. That was me paying my dues. **I then decided on taking a year out – best decision ever!** I then applied for GP training, in which I took another year out. In my experience those years out were fundamental to my development. You will be a doctor for life (hopefully!) so take the time to sit back, enjoy and appreciate your free time whilst you can. Those years out shaped my thinking, goals and personality, and helped me achieve what I wanted.

Further study

Throughout different stages in my career, I have continued with my studies at various levels:

- During my MBBS I gained a 1st in Philosophy, Medicine & Society at UCL
- During my F3 I completed my MA in History with Arabic at SOAS
- While in GP training I also completed the European Certificate of Palliative Care
- When my beloved, much-missed grandmother passed away during my GP training, I took a year out to work in A&E and I successfully passed my FRCEM Primary and ATLS; those two exams helped me transition from an A&E SHO to working as an A&E Registrar.

These external qualifications are not necessary, but they help a lot and add credence to whichever field you pursue. **Knowledge is power.**

In terms of higher educational pursuit:

- Take a look at the field in which you wish to specialise and see the qualifications needed to get ahead in that area
- Talk to the specialists or those already qualified in that area

- Ensure the opportunity comes at the right time for you and that you can carve out a work–life balance whilst managing all your responsibilities
- Do not be put off by it – it is unconventional, but it will add to your work / life. Project the decision ten years forward and see if it would benefit you then – I always think "will I regret not taking this opportunity?".

Travel

The years out have provided me the greatest mix of work and leisure. The same is true of being a locum. Take your time. I would seriously suggest everybody takes breaks from their career to help re-orient their values. I briefly lived in Egypt and was able to further my study of the Arabic language.

I found a work–life balance too: in those years I worked in Africa, South Asia and Calais for charitable ventures. Some of these trips were organised by the worldwide organisation Humanity First which is a slick, well-organised charity. It is brimming with amazing individuals who pushed me further in my career than I thought was possible and showed me opportunities I did not even know existed. I have been able to use my medical expertise abroad on multiple deployments in disaster scenarios and austere environments.

Working as a GP

Currently I work as a locum GP across multiple practices and also undertake out-of-hours and remote sessions. My workload varies from 6 to 16 sessions, but averages at about 8–10 sessions a week so far. I believe more and more of us will look to pursue a portfolio career in some way for a more flexible career in general practice in the future, to help offset the increasing stress and workload in primary care. In the future I would consider partnership if the terms were right. This would include moving abroad too. **Becoming a GP was one of the best decisions I've ever made.**

Content creation

During the Covid pandemic, I was a GPST3 and my Clinical Skills Assessment (CSA) was cancelled in February 2020. I was a part of the first cohort to sit the new Recorded Consultation Assessment (RCA) exam, which I passed first time, therefore qualifying as a GP by August 2020. It was the impetus to begin my YouTube channel in Covid. I started *so far UNSAID* to talk about working on the frontline because during the pandemic I witnessed that frontline voices were not being heard, and that was particularly true of those in the Black Asian and Minority Ethnic (BAME) communities. Coupled with my interest in race, history and religion I wanted to offer a new take on these areas. As part of this work, I have also authored some articles on Islamic history, which continues to be a topic on which I work extensively.

Publishing

I used my YouTube channel as a platform for providing free RCA resources at a time when there was little guidance available. It provided me an opportunity to offer personalised one-to-one tutorials, which I saw practically nobody else doing for the RCA, and I also provided free content which I saw nobody else doing. Then I wrote the much-needed book at the time, entitled *Essential Guide to the RCA for the MRCGP*, published by Scion Publishing Ltd.

Publishing a book is an incredible experience. To have your name as a main author on a book that can truly help people and change people's lives is amazing. Here are a few things to bear in mind:

- Be an expert in whatever you write and ensure you have thoroughly verified all your research; before writing the *Essential Guide to the RCA for the MRCGP* I had put together two brief brochures that formed a basis for a more in-depth, better-researched handbook for GP trainees
- They say any writing is re-writing. Last time I went through six drafts. It can be laborious, cumbersome and frustrating but it is always worth the effort.

Develop a book proposal before you start writing, using the following as a guideline:

1. About the author
2. Contact information
3. Title of proposed book(s)
4. Genre
5. About this topic and field
6. Brief summary
7. Target market with demographics and numbers
8. Comparative analysis presented as a table with other books in the genre with their authors and year of publishing
9. Promotion plan.

The challenges of working as a portfolio GP

When doing so many different things, it is easy to constantly feel that you're not doing enough for all your endeavours. Being a portfolio GP can be challenging to give 100% to all of one's passions. Those are the same passions that drive you. Spreading yourself thinly means working that much harder. These are the same tensions I wrote about in the limited edition *Take a Deep Breath: the diary of a junior doctor in the Covid pandemic* which went on to be in two bestseller categories on Amazon. All of these firsts helped establish me in certain areas, leading to additional opportunities such as further publishing opportunities and being interviewed by various outlets.

Advice for those considering a portfolio career

It's taken many years for me to optimise my lifestyle, commitments, leisure and family time. Daily commitment and dedication are key to building anything from the ground up. The most important thing for me is self-reflection, to plan exactly what I wish to achieve and what I want to do on a yearly basis. Every year I sit down to write out what I want to achieve financially, spiritually, physically and professionally.

Be innovative. Do you; at the same time look at what others have achieved in that field and contact them. Take on their best features. But nobody can be the best version of anyone else. **Be the best version of yourself**. It takes time, maybe years, to get there. Let your growth be natural, not forced.

There is the very real need to earn, particularly in this day and age, to give you the chance and time to seek out what is important. **Money doesn't buy happiness, but it can give you options and maybe space to make the right decisions**. Being a portfolio GP means you can choose how many hours you work and when.

I have spent my life trying to better understand the teachings of religion. Doing my best to be a practising Muslim has brought out all the good qualities in me and any shortcomings are purely my own. **Islam has provided me certainty, discipline, strength, courage and morals amongst many other things which have been sorely needed in recent difficult times.** My reading of history, my faith, the life of the Prophet Muhamad and the Holy Quran gave me the platform to base all of my decisions around.

I wish you all the best in whatever journey you choose.

6.6 Dr Julie Hammond
Healthcare advocacy, innovation and aesthetic medicine

Julie Hammond, MRCGP, DRCOG, MBBS, BSc (Hons)

- GP specialising in women's health, family planning and mental health
- Advanced aesthetic practitioner
- Passionate advocate for health equity: Kent Community NHS Foundation Trust Health Governor, Steering Group Member for the London Inspire Programme, NHS Clinical Entrepreneur, Core 20 Ambassador for NHS England, BMA EDI Advisory Group Member, member of the North Kent Maternity and Neonatal Voices Partnership and the Kent and Medway LMNS Equity and Equality Oversight Group, Trustee of West Kent Mind and chair of diversity, equity and inclusion subcommittee, Director of Events of Black Female Doctors UK and a UN Women UK delegate

Journey into medicine

Growing up I always had clear ambitions of becoming a doctor, but this goal seemed just beyond my reach. As the eldest child of first-generation migrants, I encountered several challenges navigating the education system, including attending a failing secondary school and struggling to obtain work experience to demonstrate my passion for medicine. In the early years of my studies and medical career this led me to struggle with imposter syndrome, which often made me doubt my abilities and question whether I belonged in the medical field. This feeling was compounded by my initial academic setbacks, such as when I received grades of C, D, D and E in my AS levels, which forced me to take an unplanned gap year to improve my grades.

I was subsequently diagnosed with dyslexia as a medical student. My specific learning difference has demanded extra effort and determination to excel in my educational pursuits and career. I have often had to make significant adaptations to how I learn and work as a clinician to manage my time and cognitive workload effectively. Navigating the demanding assignments and rigorous exams throughout medical school was challenging and required extraordinary perseverance. Despite these challenges, I earned a Psychology degree and graduated from Medicine with a distinction in clinical practice.

My struggles with dyslexia and early academic hurdles have given me a unique perspective on the importance of accessible education and support systems. These experiences have fuelled my commitment to advocating for an inclusive and equitable healthcare system reflective of doctors from diverse backgrounds which meets the needs of all its service users.

Early career

My career began traditionally after medical school, where I was thrust into the demanding yet rewarding world of hospital medicine as a foundation trainee. These formative years were spent gaining invaluable experience across various specialities and fine-tuning my skills in different medical settings. During this time, I was also in the midst of wedding planning and extensive home renovations, which required me to pick up extra hospital shifts to supplement my income. The relentless on-calls, night shifts and extensive hands-on training provided me with a solid clinical foundation. However, the demands of the job soon began to take their toll on both my physical and mental wellbeing. I found myself losing my passion for medicine and even considered leaving the career altogether. This period of intense workload and personal commitments prompted me to seek a more balanced and fulfilling career path. Therefore, I began exploring other careers and sources of income that I could embark upon alongside my traditional clinical training.

Aesthetic medicine

My journey into aesthetic medicine began serendipitously. I have suffered from acne and post-inflammatory hyperpigmentation since I was a teenager, and skincare and dermatological treatments have always been a crucial part of my daily regimen and something I was passionate about. Aesthetic medicine captivated me because it seamlessly blends my interests in dermatology, skincare, procedural skills and medical expertise with an artistic approach to patient care.

After discovering the field, I completed an intensive two-day training course that covered foundation and advanced Botox and dermal filler techniques. To further refine my skills, I arranged one-to-one mentoring, allowing me to master these techniques under close supervision. This hands-on experience was crucial in building my clinical skills and confidence, ensuring that I could practise safely and effectively as an advanced aesthetic practitioner.

Today, I run a successful aesthetic practice focused on achieving natural-looking results and prioritising patient safety. I have witnessed the transformative effects on clients' self-confidence, mental health and overall wellbeing that can occur as a result of improving their physical appearance. Aesthetic medicine enables me to provide holistic care that addresses both the internal and external aspects of wellbeing. As an advanced medical aesthetics practitioner, I am required to stay updated with the latest research and aesthetic advancements to ensure that I continue to provide high-quality care.

Key tips for getting started in aesthetics

- **Attend aesthetic conferences**: before investing in a course, consider attending aesthetic conferences. These events are excellent for networking, meeting like-minded professionals, and learning about new aesthetic advancements, training providers and insurers.
- **Research training providers and courses thoroughly**: ensure the course covers the aesthetic services most requested by clients and offers small group sessions to maximise cost-effectiveness and hands-on experience so you feel confident starting your aesthetics practice.
- **Join an aesthetic community**: whether through WhatsApp or Facebook groups, being part of an aesthetic community is invaluable. These communities offer encouragement, advice on challenging cases, and information on additional training and job opportunities.
- **Obtain additional medical insurance**: you will need extra insurance to cover your aesthetic practice. You can ask your training provider for recommendations on aesthetic insurers during your training.
- **Build a portfolio**: initially, unless you are fortunate enough to secure a position that provides training, consider offering free or discounted treatments to models, friends and family. High-quality before and after images and video content are crucial for attracting new clients.
- **Stay updated with trends and techniques**: the field of aesthetics is continually evolving. Regularly attending advanced training courses and workshops will keep your skills sharp and your practice up to date.
- **Create a professional online presence**: develop a professional website and maintain active social media profiles. Share

educational content, client testimonials, and before and after images to attract and engage potential clients.

- **Network with other professionals**: building relationships with other healthcare providers can lead to referrals and collaborative opportunities. Networking can also provide support and insights from experienced professionals in the field.

Getting started in aesthetics requires a substantial investment of time and money. It is not a 'get-rich quick' scheme by any means. However, if you are passionate about the field and dedicated to continuous professional development, it can be incredibly rewarding, both financially and professionally.

Health advocacy

I became pregnant during the 2020 Covid pandemic, a time when stark disparities in healthcare delivery and outcomes for individuals from BAME backgrounds, as well as marginalised communities, became glaringly apparent. These issues were particularly pertinent to me as I worked in A&E for eight months at the height of the pandemic and witnessed first-hand the realities and human experiences behind the widely reported statistics, and then subsequently went on to experience my own pregnancy loss. This personal experience fuelled my desire to empower myself and other women with the knowledge to effectively advocate for themselves and receive the care they deserve.

In pursuit of this goal, I decided to further my studies in women's health, obtaining the Diploma of the Royal College of Obstetricians and Gynaecologists (DRCOG). The DRCOG is available to any F2 doctor or above registered with the GMC or the Medical Council of Ireland (MCI) who seeks to demonstrate their interest and expand their knowledge in women's health. Prospective candidates must complete an Expression of Interest form. If accepted, they can book a place for the next available exam, which is held twice a year. There is a fee associated with booking a place to sit the exam.

My dedication to reducing health disparities has led me to seek roles beyond my clinical practice, as I have quickly realised how important it is to have a seat at the table with key decision-makers and stakeholders in order for my voice to be heard. One of the first steps I took to achieve this was applying to join the BMA's Equality, Diversity and Inclusion (EDI) committee. Here, I provide expert advice and guidance, and help to shape strategies and advocate for policy changes that facilitate equal opportunities and representation within the medical profession. Membership of the group is for two BMA sessions (two-year term).

I have also joined the London Inspire Programme as a Steering Group Member, where we focus on raising awareness and supporting the health of the Afro-Caribbean community. As a steering group member for the London Inspire Programme, I have actively contributed to initiatives aimed at improving the health of Black Londoners and reducing the health inequalities experienced by this community. This included creating the Black Health Matters social media campaign, as part of Black History Month in October 2023, to raise awareness of the common conditions which disproportionately impact the Afro-Caribbean population. I also conceived the idea for the inaugural Black Health Inequalities Summit and chaired the working group. The event attracted over 300 healthcare leaders, professionals and stakeholders, and received excellent feedback.

To further my mission of equitable healthcare, I applied for and was successfully elected as Public Health Governor for the Kent Community NHS Foundation Trust for a three-year term. In this capacity, I help to influence organisational policies to ensure inclusive healthcare delivery. I have also joined the nomination subcommittee which has allowed me to contribute to the selection of diverse leaders who drive the Trust's commitment to excellence and inclusivity.

As a 2024 Core 20 Ambassador for NHS England, I have been invited to join the North Kent Maternity and Neonatal Voices Partnership and the Kent and Medway LMNS (Local Maternal and Neonatal System) Equity and Equality Oversight Group. In these roles, I am actively collaborating with the Kent and Medway Integrated Care Board (ICB) to improve maternity care access and outcomes for women and birthing people from marginalised communities.

In addition to the above, I serve as a trustee at West Kent Mind, for which I am the Chair of the DEI Committee and a member of the Fundraising Committee. We meet on a 2–3-monthly basis, and most meetings take place in the evenings and the occasional weekend to account for the board members' work and personal commitments.

Key tips for getting started in health advocacy:

- **Volunteer with relevant organisations**: gain experience and make connections by volunteering with organisations that focus on health advocacy within your areas of interest. This can also help you understand the practical aspects of advocacy work.

- **Become a trustee**: join an organisation that aligns with your passion. Serving as a trustee can provide you with a platform to influence and contribute meaningfully to your area of interest.

- **Use your voice**: speak about the matters that are important to you. Utilise your social media platforms to raise awareness about your cause. Your voice matters and can make a significant impact.

- **Engage with policy-makers**: build relationships with local and national policy-makers. Attend public / All-Party Parliamentary Group meetings, participate in consultations and advocate for changes that support your cause.

- **Join advocacy groups and coalitions**: collaborate with established advocacy groups and coalitions, because working together can amplify your impact and provide additional resources and support.

- **Attend conferences and events in your areas of interest**: these events offer a wealth of knowledge, help you stay up-to-date, provide the opportunity to network with like-minded individuals, gain insights and make valuable connections. You can search for events within your area of interest on Eventbrite.

- **Reach out for advice and collaboration**: do not hesitate to contact those already active in the areas you are interested in. Seeking advice and discussing potential collaborations can open doors and provide invaluable guidance.

- **Create educational content**: develop and share educational materials, such as articles, videos and infographics, to inform and engage the public about your cause.

- **Consider additional training or education**: further education or training in public health, health policy, or a related field can help to deepen your understanding, enhance your advocacy skills and help you land your dream role within health advocacy.

Innovation and entrepreneurship

My role as an NHS Clinical Entrepreneur has recently become a significant aspect of my portfolio career. Recognising the need for improved health literacy among diverse populations, I am developing a pregnancy and postnatal education app that utilises cutting-edge technology. Through this app, I hope to bridge communication gaps and empower patients with the knowledge needed to take proactive steps towards a healthy pregnancy, leading to better health outcomes.

Weekly schedule

Due to the variety of my roles, no two weeks are ever the same. As a part-time salaried GP and the owner of my own aesthetic clinic, I have the flexibility to arrange my working week to fit around all of my commitments, which is invaluable to me. When needed, I can also arrange meetings in the evenings.

A typical work week can look something like this:

- Mondays and Thursdays – salaried GP role
- Tuesdays – locum GP work / meetings / admin day
- Wednesdays – off (family time)
- Fridays – aesthetic clinic / locum GP work
- Saturdays – aesthetic clinic
- Sundays – off (family time).

A diverse career path

A career in medicine is demanding and requires years of hard work and dedication. Upon graduating or completing training in your chosen speciality, it is essential to find a way to sustain your passion and motivation to ensure career longevity – we must all be aware of the physical and psychological demands and competitive nature of the career.

Increasingly, doctors are creating portfolio careers that capture their interests and drive their enthusiasm. For those considering a portfolio career in healthcare, embrace your passions and pursue roles aligning with your values. Building a diverse career requires dedication, adaptability and willingness to step outside traditional boundaries. Seek mentorship, engage with your community, and commit to continuous learning and professional development. These elements are fundamental to staying motivated and inspired in your medical career.

A portfolio career offers the flexibility to explore different facets of healthcare and find areas where you can make the most significant impact. You can integrate your various interests and skills, and create a bespoke, dynamic and fulfilling professional journey that can enhance your work satisfaction, prevent burnout, and ensure that you remain passionate about your work throughout your career.

Conclusion

My career path has been a blend of clinical practice, advocacy, innovation and aesthetic medicine, all driven by my desire to maintain a healthy work–life balance and make a commitment to reducing health disparities and improving healthcare delivery. From direct patient care and organisational leadership to public health promotion and technological innovation, I aim to create a more equitable healthcare system through my work. This diverse approach allows me to tackle healthcare challenges from multiple angles, integrating clinical expertise with advocacy and innovation to develop holistic solutions that effectively address the root causes of health disparities. I am dedicated to continuing this journey, striving for a healthcare system that is equitable, inclusive and accessible for everyone.

6.7 Dr Nigel Giam
Medical education and entrepreneurialism

Interviewed by Cansu Ozdemir

> **Nigel Giam, MBBS (Hons), MRCP, MRCGP (Distinction), DRCOG, DCH, DFFP, BSc, PGCertMedEd**
>
> - GP and lead training programme director for the St Mary's scheme, based in north-west London
> - GP tutor and seminar lead at King's College London, primarily teaching final-year medical students
> - GP Training Programme Director and works in the Centre for Pharmacy Postgraduate Education (CPPE)
> - Runs MRCGP preparation courses
> - Mentor for doctors who are having problems with GMC revalidation

How it all began

According to Dr Giam, around 20 years ago there seemed to be a very fixed 'traditional model' of general practice; the expectation was to work as a salaried GP with a view to partnership at the practice. After graduating medical school, he didn't think he would develop a portfolio career, or even qualify as a GP in the first place! He worked as a medical registrar at St Thomas' hospital after completing the core medical training programme. He felt 'swept along' with everyone else in a hamster wheel.

"After getting my MBBS, it was one of the best days of my life, but when I got my MRCGP, I felt like it was one of the worst days of my life because I felt like I'm caught in this bubble which I can't burst" and as a result, he suffered from burnout. Dr Giam was a medical registrar for around six months between the years 1999 and 2000, before deciding that it was not for him. After realising this, he started his three-year GP Training Programme and gained his CCT during 2003.

Dr Giam has always been interested in teaching: his mum was a primary school teacher and he started teaching when he was in his final year at Guy's, King's and St Thomas' School of Medicine (GKT), teaching first-year students and delivering tutorials. After qualifying as a GP, he joined the local RCGP faculty education board. This culminated in him leading and delivering membership courses, because at the time he believed that there were not many successful ones out there; he requested to pilot a different course and revamp the delivery. This new pilot course became well known and so he set up his own medical education business to deliver MRCGP teaching.

Dr Giam recounts how medical education was initially meant to be a hobby. However, this increasingly became a passion, which then evolved into being the main focus of his portfolio career – his clinical commitment has now dropped to just 10% of his overall workload. Primarily now he works as a medical educator for undergraduate medical students at GKT, a GP Training Programme Director for the St Mary's GPVTS and a clinical tutor for clinical pharmacists on the CPPE programme. Alongside these commitments, he spends much of his time on his own medical education company (Mentormeducation) that specialises in exam preparation for the MRCGP.

Breakdown of workload

- Dr Giam's medical education company takes up 6–7 sessions a week; this involves running online and face-to-face written and practical exam courses for the MRCGP, in addition to 1–2 mentoring sessions
- His role as a GP tutor requires on average 1 session every fortnight
- His GP Training Programme Director role requires 2–3 sessions a week
- The role of a clinical tutor at the CPPE takes 3 sessions a month
- Dr Giam works on average 4 clinical sessions a month as a GP locum.

For those who wish to get into similar roles specifically within medical education, Dr Giam has some advice:

- **Speak to your GP practice** – do they have space to accommodate students undertaking the postgraduate certificate in medical education (PGCertMedEd), for example?
- **Contact the primary care department leads of the medical school** – they might have opportunities for either remote or face-to-face teaching.

The pros and cons of a portfolio career

One of the highlights of having a portfolio career is that it will give you the flexibility to construct a schedule that revolves around your interests. However, the flipside to this is that unlike a typical job, you may not have a guaranteed schedule to your week, which can be a *"little bit unnerving when you don't know where you're going to be working, or what you're going to be doing".*

A portfolio career to many is seen as having a lot of different interests and, whilst this is true, Dr Giam believes it goes much deeper than this and is about *"having the autonomy to choose what you are interested in and give yourself the flexibility to make an informed choice about where you want your career to go".*

One of the disadvantages to a portfolio career is that you may not have continuity with the patient: you only have a *"dip into their narrative"* for a short amount of time and *"never know where that narrative goes".* Dr Giam believes that a great aspect of general practice is about continuity and having ongoing relationships with your patients: *"you just can't underestimate the power of human touch".*

Dr Giam's advice to his trainees is to jump into the deep end; think about *"spreading your wings and getting as much exposure to different types of specialities as you can".* For those who qualified over 20 years ago, many felt the pressure to keep climbing up a ladder within the hierarchy of medicine and aiming for that consultancy post, which can be draining. Dr Giam is an advocate for not just *"jumping into this hierarchy, but actually making an informed choice"* and this is the biggest advantage of having a portfolio career.

The biggest challenge that someone would face now if they wanted to start a portfolio career is finding the time to develop interests whilst still in training. If we look at general practice as the core specialty where we're developing a portfolio career, then it's a very busy year to fit in other interests. Ultimately, Dr Giam believes it comes down to just how passionate you are about what you want to do, knowing what you envisage your portfolio career to be for yourself and why you want to pursue it.

Advice for starting a portfolio career

It is important to ask yourself what you want from a portfolio career: is it the work–life balance? Is it because you don't want to burn out just doing general practice? Is it financially driven? What is the incentive for having a portfolio career? Dr Giam has seen trainees who are spread so thinly that they don't actually enjoy their career because they've been pulled in too many different directions.

It is important to think about how to fit your interests realistically around your working schedule. Dr Giam believes that medical education is one of the easier interests to incorporate because there are so many opportunities as a GP trainee to teach, so it can fit into your working schedule, whereas the other aspirations require a lot of additional training outside of a general practice model. You may need to sacrifice your annual leave to do this since the courses won't be covered by study leave as they are not core to general practice; NHS England makes it very clear that non-GP courses won't be covered by study leave as they are not mandatory courses but aspirational ones. This can be a major challenge to trying to develop a portfolio career.

If you are going into a field such as aesthetic or sports medicine, then there is an expectation that you get the appropriate accreditation or qualifications for that area. However, for medical education, it is possible to do an MSc in medical education which focuses on the theoretical aspect, but what Dr Giam thinks is more important (and what's recognised as accredited training) is how much delivery of medical education you have actually done, whether that's *"at an undergraduate level, working as a seminar leader, or as a GP tutor or at a postgraduate level as a trainer"*.

For those wanting to start a portfolio career, Dr Giam suggests asking yourself three questions:

1.   Why do you want a portfolio career?

A five-year planning exercise is recommended in this context – making an informed choice as to what a portfolio career involves rather than just being attracted by the notion of a portfolio career is important.

2.   What does that involve on a day-to-day basis for you?

It is important to prioritise what you feel you would want to develop within that portfolio and how you are going to fit this around your training as a practising doctor.

3.   How will you be able to practically develop your skills to become a portfolio GP?

Is a portfolio career something that you can develop as an undergraduate? Will you have the finances to attend these additional courses?

One of the things about having a portfolio career is that you need to invest in that portfolio – it's like any investment: *"If you're going to think about a portfolio career, you need to be thinking about why you want it, how you're going to prioritise the different aspects of it and how much time you're willing to give to each of them".*

Dr Giam explains that you can only truly develop a portfolio career once you have obtained your CCT in your chosen speciality. Avoid spreading yourself too thinly, being interested in so many things but actually not focusing on why you're recruited to the GP programme (to become a GP, or to work as GP if you have completed your training). Ultimately, if you are not a GP first and foremost, you'll not get any of those other aspects to your portfolio. It is good to have aspirations, but ultimately you have to have an anchor and need to make sure that it is really well rooted because if it is not, then your portfolio is going to drift off in different directions.

In five years' time, the landscape of general practice will have most likely changed again: we are heading to a point where it's very much about just seeing patients: *"getting them in and out through the door"* and not building that rapport with them. For Dr Giam, it remains important to invest in continuity, *"Whatever you decide to do, whether it's with patients or it's medical education, there has to be a theme of continuity".*

As for everyone in healthcare, it's been a challenging time recently for Dr Giam; his five-year plan was to develop his membership course and this was going well until the pandemic started and the membership exam had to change – he therefore had to evolve and keep up with the change. He would like to get back into Objective Structured Clinical Examination (OSCE) teaching, as he finds teaching undergraduates very fulfilling because students are very much open to learning.

He is still unsure about whether he will change career paths again; he is still passionate about teaching but does not particularly enjoy remote teaching. If medical education returns to more face-to-face teaching, Dr Giam believes that he will carry on: *"I like conversations and I think if you can't have a conversation because you're being compromised remotely, whether that's within education or in a clinical context, then it is something I don't feel particularly passionate about. So I don't really know where I'm going to be in five years".*

Dr Giam believes that portfolio careers will always be part of his future and may become more common, but won't be *"the future".* He feels a portfolio career should have continuity at its core instead of a *"little bit of this and a little bit of that"* with no continuity whatsoever.

Summary

In conclusion, being a portfolio GP is rewarding because you are able to merge your interests into your job and have a sense of freedom when it comes to your timetable. This may be the future of general practice, but it is important to remember that one of the main reasons for undertaking a career as a GP is for that sense of patient continuity which may become impacted in such a portfolio career. Make sure that your work as a GP comes first and think realistically about how you will be able to fit in other passions.

6.8 Dr Lee David
Cognitive behavioural therapy and author

Interviewed by Dr Vanessa Otti

Lee David, MBBS, BSc, MA, PG Cert, MRCGP

- GP
- Accredited Cognitive Behavioural Therapy (CBT) therapist at NHS Practitioner Health
- Red Whale mental health course director
- Author, educator and speaker

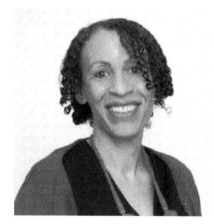

Dr David is a GP by background and was inspired to also become a cognitive behavioural therapist due to her interest in people and their stories. She combines her passions through her roles as a clinician and CBT therapist with NHS Practitioner Health and Mental Health Course Director at Red Whale. In 2008, Dr David founded her educational company '10 Minute CBT', which offers CBT training to healthcare professionals, teachers and social workers. She is also the author of four books about CBT, mental health and wellbeing, with a further three books in the works. Dr David also speaks at wellbeing events, such as 'Self-care in 10 Minutes', a talk with Action for Happiness. Dr David's work is not only transformative but immensely practical.

General practice

Dr David has worked as a salaried GP, locum and GP partner. She currently works as a clinician at NHS Practitioner Health.

She trained at Imperial College London Medical School and later carried out her three-year GP VTS in Oxford. The VTS had an additional six-month programme which offered funding for developing a special interest. She chose CBT as her special interest and began her Masters degree in CBT.

After completing GP training, Dr David found a role in West London which combined general practice, CBT therapy and research at Imperial College London. During this time, she also completed her Masters in CBT. The role worked out well and was the launchpad for her portfolio career. Dr David didn't have to create a portfolio career; she negotiated one job that combined all of her interests.

After completing this role, she became an accredited CBT therapist. Then Dr David moved out of London and found a salaried GP role at a practice where she later became a partner. She also went on to become a GP Trainer, and completed a postgraduate certificate in medical education.

Dr David recently decided to focus entirely on her role in mental health as a clinician with NHS Practitioner Health.

NHS Practitioner Health clinician

Covid-19 led to significant career changes for Dr David. She started working for NHS Practitioner Health (a self-referral NHS service which offers support to healthcare professionals with mental health difficulties) just before the pandemic. Dr David had planned to see her patients face-to-face before Covid-19; however, as the need for in-person consultations with mental health services is relatively low, the move to online consultations worked well and has enabled her to have a wider patient caseload across the UK.

Dr David currently works three sessions per week as an NHS Practitioner Health clinician. The role is similar to that of a GP but focuses solely on mental health. She also works approximately one session per week as a CBT therapist. In these roles, Dr David finds the opportunity to have longer consultations that focus on mental health problems in greater depth extremely rewarding and interesting. The role also offers increased flexibility.

Tips for working at NHS Practitioner Health:

- You should be a GP with an interest in mental health, a psychiatrist or an allied health professional, such as a mental health nurse or therapist.
- Vacancies within NHS Practitioner Health are advertised on the Practitioner Health website.

How to become a CBT therapist

Dr David advises that the route to becoming a CBT therapist depends on whether you want accreditation which enables you to practise independently, or if you're looking for additional CBT skills to use in your current job.

The British Association for Behavioural & Cognitive Psychotherapies (BABCP) is the accreditor for CBT therapists in the UK and Ireland, so its website (www.babcp.com) is a great resource. Courses and the core curriculum can be found on its website. The website also lists specific criteria for becoming an accredited CBT therapist.

Research and academia

Dr David's first GP role involved academic research at Imperial College London. Her research centred on incorporating CBT in 10-minute general practice consultations, and she designed educational resources that supported GPs in delivering CBT. Psychologists carried out similar research, but Dr David felt she brought a unique perspective, being a GP herself.

Dr David was offered the opportunity to continue her research through a PhD, but chose not to take this route, as she preferred to focus on clinical work and teaching. She started an educational company that focused on providing training for primary care health professionals on using CBT in routine consultations: 10 Minute CBT.

Over the years, Dr David has been involved with a range of research projects, which focused on behaviour change techniques and primary care education. These were carried out in collaboration with researchers at a number of different universities.

There are many ways to get involved with research, even without a formal or full-time role.

- You can dip in and out of research throughout your career in a range of ways; for example, a research trial, audit or quality improvement project.
- Consult your colleagues at your general practice, local hospitals and universities to discuss projects.
- The National Institute for Health and Care Research, as well as the RCGP, can offer access to datasets, funding and research networks for primary care research projects.

Only take on projects you have the time and energy to commit to!

Medical education

10 Minute CBT and Red Whale

Dr David founded 10 Minute CBT, a medical education business that offers CBT training to various professionals, from healthcare professionals to teachers and social workers. 10 Minute CBT is an innovative adaptation of evidence-based CBT techniques for short 10–30-minute sessions. The 10 Minute CBT approach is flexible and adaptable to various settings.

Dr David didn't have a background in business so starting 10 Minute CBT involved a steep learning curve. Balancing advertising and venue costs with estimates of course attendees was challenging at times, when trying to ensure there was enough demand to make a course viable. Dr David later began offering online training and providing face-to-face training commissioned by a range of educational organisations; this has reduced the administrative workload and risk associated with hosting courses. She also outsourced the administrative work and book-keeping to a support company, which has been extremely helpful in managing her own time.

Dr David recruited and trained several CBT therapists in how to deliver the training model she had developed for using CBT in primary care settings. Through the process, Dr David realised that she enjoyed teaching and clinical work above all else; she is less motivated by a managerial role. As a result, she scaled down her role at 10 Minute CBT.

Three years ago Dr David began working with a primary care education organisation called Red Whale as their course director for mental health. She works two sessions per week with Red Whale, focusing on designing resources, writing articles and delivering mental health educational content digitally and face-to-face.

Advice for working in education:

- Seek opportunities to teach in your current role, such as teaching medical students or junior doctors
- Consider completing training such as a GP Trainers course, postgraduate certificate or diploma in medical education
- Seek (and listen to) feedback every time you teach, aiming to develop your knowledge and skills in what works well for learners.

"Finding what motivates you and allowing this to evolve is key to maintaining a long career."

Author

Dr David began writing by approaching publishers in the primary care market with her ideas. She followed their submission process, which usually involves providing an overview of the book and sample chapters (further information is available on each publisher's website).

- Dr David first wrote *Using CBT in General Practice: the 10 minute CBT handbook* (Scion Publishing Ltd), a book aimed at GPs offering an overview of CBT and how it can be incorporated into a typical 10-minute consultation
- Dr David also published *Managing Anxiety Disorders in Primary Care* (also Scion Publishing Ltd), a practical guide on recognising and treating anxiety disorders
- *10 Minutes to Better Mental Health – A Step-by-Step Guide for Teens* (Jessica Kingsley Publishers) covers topics from managing anxiety to building self-confidence and healthy habits
- In March 2023, Dr David's book *Boosting Your Mental Wellbeing: 10 minute steps for stressed healthcare professionals using CBT and mindfulness* (also Scion Publishing Ltd) was published; this is a practical handbook designed to support wellbeing in clinicians.

Tips on how to become an author:

- Choose a subject that you are interested in and have lots of knowledge about
- Research similar work and look for a unique perspective
- Think about what your readers will hope to achieve by reading the book – it's often helpful to include practical tips and bring the text to life with case examples and stories
- Approach publishers relevant to your field.

Future career path

Dr David plans to continue her clinical and CBT therapist roles at NHS Practitioner Health and teach through Red Whale. Her other educational role as Director of 10 Minute CBT has reduced as her work with Red Whale increased, but she wants to continue both roles.

Dr David wants to write more in the future because it offers a rewarding, flexible career. She is also a speaker and plans to continue with this work in the future. She is motivated by having a voice and contributing her perspective to books and talks that will hopefully help many people.

The pros and cons of a portfolio career

Portfolio careers maintain your interest and enthusiasm; but with part-time roles and multiple commitments, you can accumulate more work as each task can potentially overrun.

With part-time work, there's the risk of becoming isolated because you're less central to any particular organisation than you would be if you worked full-time. For many of us, a sense of belonging is very important, so make an effort to connect with others and develop strong relationships.

Dr David is part of a peer learning group at NHS Practitioner Health. She makes an effort to go every month to chat with colleagues and attends the service-wide education events which are held online, and an annual face-to-face conference. Taking time to connect with colleagues in this way is invaluable, as many of the NHS Practitioner Health staff work from home.

Lastly, your overall pay might reduce when carrying out smaller, part-time roles, but on balance, making career changes that suit your interests and offer more freedom should be positive.

Advice for those who want to start a portfolio career

Create opportunities by developing your skills, qualifications and experience in different areas. With each new skill, new options open up for you. At times, you might not know what the possibilities are going to be. Dr David didn't initially plan on working for NHS Practitioner Health and Red Whale. She gained a PG Certificate in medical education as part of her GP Training role and mental health skills from her interest in CBT. So, when Red Whale contacted Dr David with an opportunity, she already had the credentials for educational work, which she knew she would enjoy.

Dr David's portfolio career developed through her genuine interests. After completing her Masters CBT and accreditation, she thought about how she could continue practising as a CBT therapist and share her experience with others. So, she developed her training model and achieved her PG Cert. Then she thought, *"how am I doing with this training? I believe in it and feel like I have more to say. So how can I deliver that?"* Then she set up the 10 Minute CBT educational company and became an author and speaker.

Portfolio careers aren't necessarily for everybody; general practice can be a remarkable career in itself...

Within general practice, you can create a sense of a portfolio career by pursuing your interests without perhaps needing a separate role. Finding what motivates you and allowing this to evolve is key to maintaining a long career.

Final words about wellbeing

Dr David has learned to set boundaries to create a healthy work–life balance. Boundary setting is essential because while working with NHS Practitioner Health she sees many doctors struggling in various areas of their lives. No matter what job you do, there's always more work you can do, especially if you're thorough and conscientious. We should set boundaries around what we can realistically do, and we have to own this ourselves.

Dr David actively manages her workload by regularly reflecting, asking herself, *"how am I doing? Have I got too much work this week? Do I need to consider extending a deadline?"* It may be easy to ignore how we feel and push through difficulties, but this can cause burnout. Taking a step back and observing your experience, almost like a third person, is important when managing busy workloads; in essence, this is a way to achieve self-care.

"Whatever you're doing, make sure that your wellbeing is at the same level of importance as everything else."

6.9 Dr Henrietta Hughes
Giving patients a voice

Interviewed by Manas Soni

> **Henrietta Hughes, OBE, MA (Oxon), MBBS, FRCGP, SFFMLM, DRCOG, DFFP**
>
> - Locum GP
> - Non-executive director of the South Central Ambulance Service
> - NHS appraiser
> - Chair of the children's charity Childhood First
> - School governor
> - Member of the Honours committee at the Cabinet Office

Dr Hughes was previously appointed as the NHS National Guardian (where she introduced Freedom to Speak Up Guardians across the NHS) and a medical director at NHS England. She was made a FRCGP during 2019, honoured with an officer of the Order of the British Empire (OBE) medal in the Queen's New Year Honours List in 2020, and was awarded Senior Fellowship of the Faculty of Medical Leadership and Management during 2021.

Typical working week

Before Dr Hughes accepted the Patient Safety Commissioner role, a typical week would involve working as a GP for 2–3 days. Dr Hughes typically spends one day a week as the non-executive director of the South Central Ambulance Service; in addition, this role involves a significant amount of reading prior to meetings. Her roles as a school governor, chair at Childhood First and appraiser usually require half a day in total each week. The honours committee requires biannual attendance at meetings.

How it all began

Dr Hughes' career as a portfolio GP was unplanned; she was initially looking to pursue a career in obstetrics and gynaecology. As a medical student, she shadowed junior doctors in an IVF clinic in the USA over two summers. However, she retrained as a GP due to a lack of flexibility in the location of available obs and gynae rotations.

Dr Hughes was interested in leadership roles as early as medical school. She undertook courses at the NHS Leadership Academy which developed her collaborative and patient-centred leadership style. Early on in her career she engaged in quality improvement (QI). She made it a priority to listen to colleagues' concerns and queries relating to the management of patient care. Once she led a few QI projects acting on issues highlighted by her colleagues, she could harmonise teams that were not functioning to their maximum potential due to structural and practical issues. These skills were further developed when she ran a course for newly qualified GPs. She highlighted that from her early experiences *"bringing people together to discuss problems"*, that the *"relentless monitoring"* of policies was required to find solutions.

Whilst Dr Hughes was the lead appraiser for a Primary Care Trust (PCT), she brought together five leads of local PCTs to develop the most effective management strategies. Each PCT had its own unique strengths and weaknesses demonstrated by its performance. The leads discussed various methods they used to achieve their targets and this *"pooled expertise"* was used to create effective management strategies.

Dr Hughes was concerned that the change she instituted in this role could be undone, so when the role of deputy medical director at the North Central London Cluster was advertised, she decided to apply. She was therefore able to continue the performance-based teamwork style of management. Her role as deputy medical director was cut short after her boss took personal leave and she was promoted to acting medical director; she then applied to be a Medical Director at the newly-formed NHS England, making her responsible for roughly 3000 GPs in the North Central and East London. Her passion for improving the quality of care for patients, previously demonstrated by her involvement in QI and as the deputy director, gave her the relevant experience and background to thrive in this role.

As the National Guardian for the NHS, Dr Hughes set up 'Freedom to Speak Up' across England, managing 50 000 patient and staff wellbeing cases. Given her passion for such issues, she found this role highly rewarding despite its considerable commitment. She has recently been appointed as the first Patient Safety Commissioner to improve the safety of medicines and medical devices. This appointment was made following Baroness Cumberlege's *First Do No Harm* report during 2022, highlighting the issues related to using Primodos, sodium valproate and pelvic mesh. Her role is to promote patient safety and to ensure that patients have more of a voice.

Things to consider when working as a portfolio GP

Organisation is key for a portfolio GP, given the various tasks in a typical week. Planning and allowing for allocated time for the preparation and pre-reading of meeting documents is vital to make the most of the limited time available for each commitment. Dr Hughes stressed that in a leadership role, being prepared and up-to-date for each event is important to ensure that her management strategies can be implemented. She keeps a single diary for all work and personal responsibilities to stay on top of each commitment.

She mentioned that there were several *"problems which needed to be fixed"* within the GP system, and whenever an opportunity arose in the form of a job which addressed those problems, she applied for the role. Dr Hughes stressed the importance of seizing opportunities when they occurred (especially when they align with your personal aims and goals) and she feels this is vital to developing a portfolio career.

Dr Hughes' drive to put patients first and working collaboratively with patients and healthcare professionals has shaped the trajectory of her career and helped her excel in her various commitments.

Her final piece of advice for those early in their careers was to write a 'personal business plan' highlighting factors such as career aims, ideal career length and location of employment. This plan will help provide a basis for career decisions throughout one's lifetime. There should also be an overall goal to strive for.

She stressed the importance of doing something you have a genuine interest in, as we all have *"limited time but unlimited energy"*; when pursuing something you are passionate about, it does not *"take much energy"*. For example, given her drive to improve patient wellbeing, roles such as chairing Childhood First and the National Guardian are highly rewarding for Dr Hughes. She highlighted that essential skills can be developed through free online courses and engaging with societies and opportunities when they arise, even as a student.

Conclusion

Dr Hughes' main advice was *"to do things you find interesting"* and to follow your passions to make working as enjoyable as possible. She also mentioned that her range of paid and voluntary roles initially *"didn't appear to connect to each other"*, but as she progressed in her career, these collective experiences were *"invaluable"*.

6.10 Dr Usman Sajjad
Sports medicine

Interviewed by Dr Ahmed Al-Wizni

Usman Sajjad ('Dr Uz'), MBChB, MPhil, MRCGP

- Salaried GP
- Sports doctor to some of the biggest names in boxing and the Ultimate Fighting Championship
- Medical director for a Covid testing company
- Main clinician for a testosterone company which treats men with hypogonadism

Where it all began

Dr Uz explained that his career in sports medicine began after completing a one-year sports diploma. *"I decided to take an FY3 year to really figure out what I wanted to do, even though I pretty much had an idea in FY2. I completed my sports medicine diploma during 2022 and gained more clinical experience and exposure. More clinical experience is always a good thing."* He feels that achieving a diploma opened doors to many ventures in sports medicine. He first worked for Everton Women's FC between 2017 and 2018; however, although he was a supporter and fan of Everton FC, he decided football was not the sport he wanted to work in. *"I more enjoyed treating athletes with different, perhaps more serious injuries, such as head injuries."* Hence, he decided to change direction, which led to working for Widnes Vikings Rugby league between 2018 and 2020.

Dr Uz attributes his success in sports medicine to the launch of his podcast 'The Doctor Uz Podcast' in 2020; he interviewed people from various industries, from authors to physiotherapists. *"The podcast really helped me build connections with many people in different sectors of work."* One of the episodes features a special guest who was Tyson Fury's massage therapist. They kept in contact, which eventually led to Dr Uz being recommended by him to Tyson. *"Tyson would often complain about not being able to get GP appointments, then one day I was recommended by his massage therapist just before the third Deontay Wilder fight. They wanted joint injections to the elbow which I said I can do, as well as some Covid testing as they were flying to Vegas for the fight and needed it."* Dr Uz also explained that he built a friendship with Tyson Fury and his team due to clinical work he did free of charge. *"Fury asked to pay me, but I refused and told him it was just an honour to work with you* and help you out." "I also said money's not an issue for me, and he must've liked that as he laughed, and we were friends from then on." Dr Uz would later sign with Tyson and the rest of the Fury team, including Tommy Fury. He recommends doing "favours and the favours will pay you back."

Dr Uz would later sign with other athletes such as Joseph Parker, Isaac Lowe, Anthony Fowler, Nathan Gorman, Conor Benn and Joe Cordina, and become the resident doctor for the gym that hosts UFC fighters Paddy 'The Baddy' Pimblett and Molly McCann. With such an impressive portfolio of fighters, Dr Uz aspires to become the most renowned and sought-after sports doctor in combat sports.

It is crucial to consider the not so nice aspects to working with celebrity patients. Whilst working with Tommy Fury he was the target of abuse. "The hate and abuse I received when I pulled Tommy Fury out of the fight because of his broken ribs was crazy." Tommy Fury suffered a rib fracture prior to an upcoming fight, and Dr Uz felt it was not safe for him to engage in that fight. This triggered angry fans, causing them to leave hateful comments on Dr Uz's social media platforms. "You really have to be careful about what you say in the public eye."

Three top tips from Dr Uz for building a portfolio career centred around sports medicine

1. Network, network, network – put yourself out there and build connections with people in the field or close to athletes you want to work with. Dr Uz helped Fury and his team with their Covid-19 jabs, just because he respected and admired him, without asking for anything in return. This was a key catalyst to kickstarting their working relationship.

2. Follow your passions and adapt – Dr Uz had a passion for boxing and combat sports, being an amateur boxer himself, and so he immediately fitted in. The boxing world is completely different to medicine: you may be in the limelight and you may have to defend your decisions. Adapting to this new pressured environment is key.

3. Take the initiative to try new things – Dr Uz started a podcast during lockdown without the slightest idea that it could lead to him working with the boxing champion Tyson Fury. So, think about what you could get started with working on – you never know what could happen!

Working in general practice

Alongside his sports medicine career, Dr Uz also works as a salaried GP Wednesday to Friday at a small practice; *"There are only two GPs at our practice – me and one other"*. When asked about his clinical practice, he referred to location being an important factor for him. *"I work in a deprived area, which often means I get to see very different pathologies."*

Dr Uz prefers working as a salaried GP rather than a locum. *"I did a few months as a locum and found I was going from practice to practice and I really didn't enjoy that."* He didn't feel as if he was part of a team and felt that working as a salaried GP was a lot safer. *"They bury you if you make a mistake as a locum; as a salaried you're a lot more protected."* On the other hand, he does appreciate the positives of working as a locum, such as higher rates of pay and choosing when to work.

In the future Dr Uz would like to become a GP partner and own a GP surgery. However, he acknowledges that as a GP partner it could be more difficult to keep up with his sports medicine work as well as other commitments.

Dr Uz prides himself in working as a portfolio GP. Another special interest – hypogonadism – led to him working at a testosterone company called Alphagenix. This is a private company that works to treat men with low testosterone and primary and secondary hypogonadism. *"I worked as a GP for a private clinic and the owner who started the company asked me if I wanted to be the main clinician for it, so I accepted."* Dr Uz often refers to the importance of establishing the idea of connections and getting to know people, branching out and taking opportunities when they arise.

A typical day in the testosterone clinic consists of consultations with patients, taking blood from patients, monitoring blood tests and administering testosterone. Patients with low testosterone are treated with a testosterone replacement and can be monitored for between 6 weeks and 10 months.

When asked what particularly sparked his interest in this area of medicine, he mentioned his mother who specialises in andrology and inspires him. He also mentioned that a connection with combat sports is clear because athletes can often have low testosterone (testosterone use is banned by boxing federations). These factors led him to joining the European Andrology Society to further develop his interest.

He works at Alphagenix on Mondays and/or Tuesdays, which are often days that he also does his sports medicine side activities. He is paid per patient and per consultation. The workload varies, so some months his clinics are busy and some not so much, and this allows him to arrange his week as he sees fit. Whether that is to devote more time as a sports doctor, or as a clinician at Alphagenix, he enjoys this flexibility because he gets to shape his week to suit himself.

Dr Uz says that there are very few limitations as to what you can do as a portfolio GP: he is also the medical director for a Covid testing company located overseas. The work includes annual meetings and conducting audits, and he earns a set annual salary in this role.

At the age of 34, Dr Uz has an extremely impressive portfolio. Dr Uz advises networking and building connections with as many people in many different fields as possible. Most of his ventures were due to good connections and word of mouth: *"Get yourself out there"*. He also suggests helping people without expecting anything back. *"Do favours and the favours will pay you back eventually."*

Summary

There are many ways that a GP can work with companies or use their own special interests, such as in sports medicine. Dr Uz's main advice about creating a portfolio career is to network and build connections with as many people as possible, in as many different fields as possible – his involvement in most ventures was due to connections and word of mouth contacts. Dr Uz is a great example of the avenues that a portfolio GP can go down. The possibilities are endless; you can take your career in many different directions and there is a significant amount of freedom in how you choose to shape your portfolio career.

6.11 Dr Lavan Baskaran
GP partner, private GP, content creator and medical advisor

Interviewed by *Dr Ahmed Moussa*

> ### Lavan Baskaran, MBBS, BSc, MRCGP
>
> - Senior NHS GP principal with a private clinic in Harley Street and special interests including ADHD, ENT, diabetes, chronic kidney disease and minor surgery
> - Teaches medical students at his GP practices
> - Educates the public about a healthy lifestyle using social media
> - Medical advisor to Play Action International

Dr Baskaran's pathway to general practice was straightforward; he graduated from UCL medical school, and then completed his foundation training before GP training. He was drawn to general practice because he wanted to coordinate his time with freedom and have some flexibility in his work, in addition to the variety of day-to-day cases and varied roles of a GP. Dr Baskaran's main advice is to work hard, appreciate longer hours of training, and learn from everyone and every situation.

General practice

Dr Baskaran is a GP partner, working at two practices in London. There are roughly 20 000 patients across both practices. He spends two full working days at each practice. The first practice serves a more affluent population, whereas the second practice provides care for a less privileged population. He combines his passion for teaching with his clinical work by teaching medical students.

Dr Baskaran is absolutely satisfied with his career: *"The beauty of general practice is the ability to learn anything you like, there is a wide variety of interests that doctors can choose from, and you can always study more."* He enjoys being a part of a team, working with managers and other doctors. At his practices he feels the team is more like a family, helping and supporting each other. He also enjoys building relationships with his patients over long periods and colleagues both in the UK and abroad. Finally, general practice allows him to have a good work–life balance.

Tips for someone who wants to be a partner:

- Don't rush! The **right** partnership will present itself at the **right** time.
- Analyse the dynamics of the team you will join:
  - How does the 'senior' partner treat the junior partners: equally, or is there a difference? Is that a good or bad thing?
  - How do the partners interact or not interact with their employees? Is that how you would treat your staff members?
  - Make sure their principles align with yours, as you will be working with this team, more than you see your partner at home (!)
- Upskill – invest in yourself. Be the best clinician you can be. Develop lots of interests, so not only will you enjoy your work, and this will show in your demeanour, but you will become more employable.
- Make sure you have a firm understanding of the practice ethos, strengths and weaknesses. Think about what you could bring to the team to improve the practice and reduce the weaknesses.

Additional roles

- Private practice – Dr Baskaran works one day in a private ADHD clinic with a consultant, providing virtual consultations throughout the week if needed. He also uses this day for private work. He finds great fulfilment in seeing these patients, as he feels more could be done within the NHS for patient care.
- Social prescribing advocate – he introduced and leads in the area of social prescribing at both his GP practices. He works with companies that help people become happier and healthier in their communities through social prescribing and lifestyle changes.
- Content creator – Dr Baskaran was motivated to start a YouTube channel to promote and educate the general public about a healthy lifestyle. He works with a team of three people spending half a day every four weeks to help with the channel. He has now created medical 'life hacks' on Instagram, providing advice regarding medical conditions and a healthy lifestyle.
- Medical advisor to Play Action International. This charity improves the lives of millions of children across the world through play. He had his first experience at Butabika Mental Health Hospital in Uganda in 2015. Over the next 10 years, the plan is to support healthcare institutions in Kenya, especially

regarding children's cancers and mental health. He hopes to make a big difference in the upcoming years.

Career plans

Dr Baskaran expects to continue to work as a GP and develop all his roles. He would like to join the NHS financial advisory so that he can be involved with distributing funds. He currently undertakes similar work at AstraZeneca and Novo Nordisk.

Advice for starting a portfolio career

- **Undertake additional qualifications:** *"If you want to be more confident in your knowledge and abilities you should do other qualifications."*

Dr Baskaran completed the MRCP part I and II, and the MRCS-ENT exams, and these help in his work as a GP due to the variety of cases he sees. In 2022 he completed training in ADHD at King's College London and he is now in the process of completing a PG Cert in gender identity at the University of London and the Royal College of Physicians. *"I love to learn. People will trust you more if you have other qualifications in your area of specialism."*

- **Make the most of situations and seize opportunities:** *"Ask to perform some procedures and do not hesitate to take the opportunity to learn from others. For example, do not step back from performing minor surgery, sutures."*

Creating variety can prevent you becoming bored and demotivated. With so many roles available, why limit yourself? You can be a trainer, examiner or researcher and can develop a special interest.

Summary

Dr Baskaran is a senior NHS GP principal with special interests in ADHD, ENT, diabetes, CKD and minor surgery, and he is passionate about medical education. He has developed additional roles in private practice, social prescribing, content creation and medical advisory work. The MRCP and MRCS-ENT exams have significantly benefited his clinical work. His main piece of advice for creating a portfolio career is to develop your skill set because this not only improves the confidence you and others have in your abilities, but also creates opportunities for the future.

6.12 Dame Clare Gerada
Leadership

Interviewed by *Dr Pavan Marwaha*

> **Dame Clare Gerada, MBBS, DBE, PRCGP, FRCP (Hon), FRCPsych**
>
> - NHS GP partner with specialist interests in mental health, drug, alcohol and gambling addiction, and the management of healthcare professionals with mental health
> - Chair and President of the RCGP – the second woman in its 70-year history to hold both leadership roles
> - Extensively published author.

Dame Gerada works as an NHS GP partner who has had many roles and accolades during her career. Most notably, at the time of writing Dame Gerada is the Chair and President of the Royal College of General Practitioners (RCGP) and is the second woman in its seventy-year history to hold both leadership roles: Chair and President.

In addition to her public recognition awards, Dame Gerada was also City Woman of the Year (2012), nominated for BBC Woman of the Year (2013) and awarded other accolades for her work, including the *BMJ* Mental Health Service of the year for the Practitioner Health Programme (2018).

Despite never holding any paid academic role, Dame Gerada has published extensively in peer-reviewed, non-peer-reviewed, mainstream and trade press publications. She has contributed chapters to the works of others and has written and edited three books, the most recent being *Beneath the White Coat: doctors, their minds and mental health*. She also is a regular blog writer for the *BMJ*.

How it all began

During 1982 Dame Gerada qualified from University College and Middlesex School of Medicine, now UCL Medical School. She then went on to complete her medical training. After initially training in psychiatry, Dame Gerada made the transition to general practice, starting her career at the Hurley Clinic where she has been senior partner since 1992. Within general practice, she has also been a GP trainer – including training GPs who were on the induction and returner scheme (this scheme enables GPs who have previously been on the GMC's GP Register and on the NHS National Performers List, to safely return to general practice following a career break; the scheme also supports the safe introduction of GPs who have qualified outside the UK and have no previous NHS GP experience).

Involvement in mental health

Since late 2019 Dame Gerada has been the lead for the Primary Care Gambling Service – a pioneering service bridging the gap between current third sector services and primary care. This service aims to increase the number of gamblers accessing treatment and improve the knowledge about gambling amongst the primary care community. Within this role she leads a team of clinicians, including general practitioners, mental health and general nurses, therapists and a consultant psychiatrist. She dedicates a significant amount of time and effort to this role: *"Setting up a brand new service during the pandemic was hard, with numbers entering the service constantly increasing"*.

While reflecting on her involvement in mental health provisions, Dame Gerada stated that *"General practice is the number one speciality to redefine yourself every few years"*. Whilst working as a psychiatry registrar (specialising in addiction), Dame Gerada gained her experience and transferable skills which helped her set up the Primary Care Gambling Service: *"I ran a homeless service for intravenous drug users, then set up a shared care service. I was asked to do the same for gambling to shorten the gap in referral times, by creating an intermediary and causing a paradigm shift (where GP refers patient to specialist). The only experience prior to this in gambling was as an undergraduate medical student in psychology where I learned about intermittent variable reinforcement"*. Since the inception of the service, Dame Gerada has become an expert advisor on a major research project undertaken by a group attached to Queen Mary University of London. She has also been asked by NHS England to explore future treatment services.

Tips about developing a career in treating mental health and substance abuse:

- See the need in the consulting room and explore how you can develop your skills
- Obtain a certificate developed by the RCGP in substance misuse
- Attend conferences on mental health and substance abuse.

Involvement in presidency

In November 2021, Dame Gerada became President of the RCGP. She has had an extensive history with the Royal College: *"Initially, I had no idea who they (the College) were, but I took the RCGP College exam in 1995. GPs were not initially involved in drug provisions. I, in a group of four, wanted to work together to create a primary care strategy but needed the RCGP to legitimise the work we were doing. I approached the president-elect back then, David Haslam. I asked if we could develop a training programme, start badging some statements like 'drug users have a right to care like anyone else'. I was so overwhelmed by his kindness and positivity that I got involved in the College Council for faculty work and never left since"*. Dame Gerada was the second female chair in its history and the first for over 50 years. Her role included chairing a council of 60-plus members, as well as leading the direction and strategy, and being the figurehead of the professional body. Her achievements as chair included developing the 2020 vision for general practice, obtaining governmental and professional agreement to extend GP training from three to four years, and leading the response to the 2012 NHS Act.

Tips about getting into leadership positions in professional colleges:

- Get the membership for the professional College you want to join
- Join the professional College's (most likely RCGP) faculty – it will enable you to meet like-minded individuals
- Get involved and get stuck in! You can also join your local medical committee.

Reflecting on the past

Despite her many roles and accolades, Dame Gerada did not plan any of them, with her motto being *"say yes and figure it out after"*. She acknowledged the worries she had when starting off in her career and feeling like she got the balance wrong between her career and family life. A key reflection on career was *"the more you do, the more opportunities come"*.

- Take some time off during the week and spend it with those you love – she wished she took *"a Friday afternoon off and Monday morning so that I could spend more time with my children"*.
- Make or join a support group so that you do not feel alone, especially during the beginning of your career.

The future

Dame Gerada hopes to add more to her already incredible career. Her future aspirations include:

- becoming more involved in writing
- potentially getting into politics
- meeting the next generation of doctors and students to see how she can support them.

Advice about portfolio careers

Dame Gerada provided her own definition of the term portfolio careers: *"A number of roles and responsibilities which make up the totality of me"*, with the word portfolio meaning *"flexibility and enjoyment"*.

With that in mind, Dame Gerada offered many words of advice for individuals wanting to pursue a portfolio career:

- Do something you enjoy – *"Life is too short to be doing something you don't like"*.
- Learn your craft and see what positive changes you can make – *"See where your craft takes you. By undertaking these roles, I have developed my craft and always worked hard and saw what in the consultation room needed sorting out"*.
- Get involved – Dame Gerada mentions advice focusing on general practice: *"The generalism of the speciality allows us to get involved in anything. Explore what comes next. As GPs we know how to handle risk"*.
- Believe in yourself – *"Follow your nose. When people say you can't do something, you can. Don't expect anyone to notice your hard work or give you a pat on the shoulder"*.

Summary

Dame Gerada's career has stemmed from her early passions. While being a GP, she was able to curate a multifaceted portfolio of her roles and responsibilities which have aligned with her work in mental health and leadership. After spending time in the mental health sector, RCGP presidency and as a GP partner, she is excited to see what the future has in store for her transition to writing (and possibly politics). To summarise, Dame Gerada's message is simple: do what you enjoy, find your niche, and say yes to opportunities.

6.13 Dr Nicola Elliott
Medical education, medical officer and diving medical referee

Interviewed by Dr Gireesha Verma

Nicola Elliott, BSc (Hons), MBBS, MRCGP, PGCert Clin Ed, Diploma Diabetes Care, Diploma in Child Health, Standard Underwater Medicine Course

- Locum GP
- Educationalist
- Medical referee for divers
- Medical officer for a girls' boarding school
- Volunteer with Refugee Education UK

Dr Elliott's portfolio career is a kaleidoscope of her interests and passions. She was *"attracted to GP… due to the fact that there's so much variety and opportunity to develop a portfolio career"*. Dr Elliott relishes the challenges of her diverse vocation which also allows her to spend more time with her family.

How it all began

After graduating from UCL Medical School in 2001, Dr Elliott completed what is now known as foundation training followed by GP training, gaining her CCT in 2006. She was always inclined towards exploring different professional opportunities. After consideration of the numerous benefits to a portfolio career (variety, flexibility, work–life balance, ability to be your own boss), followed by a final nudge from professional coaching sessions, she decided to pursue this path. She has not looked back since.

General practice

Dr Elliott has worked as a GP partner, salaried GP and locum GP. After qualifying she initially started work as a GP partner, but after a few years, she relocated to a new partnership. During 2013 she completed a diploma in Diabetes Care at Warwick University, after which she was appointed as the clinical lead for diabetes at the practice. As the practice expanded and developed, Dr Elliott became a salaried GP; while the role still entailed being involved in management decisions and meetings (as she had been a partner previously), there was specific time allotted for it. She reminisces that the shift came with mixed feelings (fewer hassles, no worry about staff recruitment / appraisal, but she also missed the role of being a partner). She started as a locum GP during September 2022 and currently works 1–2 clinical sessions a week.

Dr Elliott's advice on general practice:

- **Team rapport**: *"Join a team who have a coffee meeting every day"*. Working in a practice is like a long-term investment with the practice partners. Partners getting on well with each other is beneficial and leads to a conducive work environment.

- **GP partner**: Dr Elliott mentions work flexibility and being your own boss as two advantages of being a GP partner. Better salary also used to be a bonus, but that is less true in recent times.

- **Salaried GP**: look for a practice which will allow you to do your special interest, as a bit of variety helps prevent burnout. Ask about opportunities for special interest roles, which are generally easier to do in bigger or training practices.

- **Locum GP**: the challenges of locum roles involve not knowing the practice fully (if not a regular locum GP) and therefore having less understanding of how the practice functions. Dr Elliott emphasises that a locum GP strives to earn the trust of people (colleagues as well as patients) in every new practice, whereas in long-term roles people may feel that they can trust that doctor more (which is something she misses about being a regular GP).

Medical education

Dr Elliott is a really passionate medical educationalist, to whom it *"feels like working with young doctors who are very enthusiastic and are the future of the NHS"*.

"A GP colleague in my practice helped me realise that this is where my passion lies", says Dr Elliott, and she began cultivating an interest in it from her early years as a GP. It was extremely important for her to find working environments with teaching opportunities.

Further training led her to become a clinical supervisor for FY2 trainees and a clinical and educational supervisor for GP trainees. She also completed a Postgraduate Certificate in medical education during her training to become a supervisor.

As being an educationalist is one of her priorities, Dr Elliott mentions *"when switching from a salaried to a locum role, I was worried that I might not get to continue with a teaching role"*. However, she was able to find many teaching opportunities.

Shortly after resigning from her salaried job, Dr Elliott came across an advert for the role of Primary Care Facilitator at the University of Buckingham, which she applied for; she was subsequently appointed, and has been in this role since September 2022. The role is seasonal (3–4 months per year) and involves 2 days' structured teaching on communication and consultation skills for medical students on their clinical placements in primary care. She also examines at medical student OSCEs.

Dr Elliott recollects that during the 2022 summer holidays she was volunteering for the Commonwealth Games as a GP for the athletes and during her time there she met the lead for Case-Based Learning (CBL) at Warwick University who was also volunteering as a GP. She spoke about her passion for medical education and was subsequently informed about an opening for the role of a CBL facilitator at Warwick University and was encouraged to apply. She applied and was appointed! She currently facilitates small group CBL across all phases of medical school teaching. Dr Elliott explains that her role is "*to facilitate this and prompt learning areas if needed, or prompt further discussion, rather than to teach directly*".

Recently Dr Elliott has been appointed as an Enhanced Educational Supervisor, which is a new role being piloted. She explains that this role is for experienced trainers who are leaving general practice. They don't qualify to be educational supervisors, but their experience and skills can be utilised to support struggling trainees with extra tutorials as well as specific tailored help and guidance.

Dr Elliott's advice for roles in medical education:

- **Additional qualifications**: PGCert Medical Education is very important and is a requirement for certain teaching roles in medical education. Even in roles where it might not be an essential requirement, it will be an advantage when applying for teaching roles.
- **Balancing act**: although teaching roles are not as well-paid as clinical roles, the working hours are better, with no clinical uncertainty and no out-of-hours commitments. That said, during summer holidays there is no teaching so more locum work might be needed to supplement income.

Medical officer

Dr Elliott has previously served as a medical officer for a girls' boarding school for one session a week as part of her partner role and subsequent salaried role as a GP. The role involved providing medical care for a girls' school, PSHE (personal, social, health and economic) education, contraception and sexual health education, as well as working with nurses and teachers to help with pastoral support for the school. She found the role really rewarding and one of a kind, seeing the schoolgirls grow through their formative years (11–18 years), building up a trusting relationship with them and supporting them through various issues when their parents weren't close by.

Dr Elliott's advice for the role of medical officer in a school:

- **Explore**: ask about these roles, especially when working as a salaried GP. You might find them where there are boarding schools.
- **Out-of-hours**: you might receive queries (by text message, for example) from the nurses at any time for advice about urgent issues.

Diving medical referee

Dr Elliott learned to scuba dive at university, during which she found out that there were doctors with a special interest in diving medicine. After further research she completed a dive medicine course at the Institute of Naval Medicine. Since 2008 she has been a qualified licensed diving medical referee. She is a member of the UK Diving Medical Committee (UKDMC; www.ukdmc.org) and is registered on the diving medical referees' register. Diving medical referees undertake medical testing and verify divers' fitness to dive. There are also some other specialisations related to diving medicine (also known as undersea and hyperbaric medicine) which include managing diving injuries and medical issues of occupational divers (e.g. deep-sea divers, oil rig divers). The UKDMC holds a two-day conference for members every other year for updates and social events. It also has online forums to discuss cases with more experienced and specialist doctors.

Dr Elliott's advice for the role of diving medical referee:

- **Diving**: having a diving qualification is a prerequisite
- **Indemnity**: additional indemnity is required
- **Seasonal with out-of-hours**: although the work is seasonal (more work during diving season), doctors might need to respond (by emails / phone calls / remote / in-person consultations) at any time for advice regarding fitness or other urgent concerns.

Volunteering

During 2020, Dr Elliott started volunteering with Refugee Education UK (www.reuk.org) as a mentor in English and Maths for unaccompanied asylum seekers (mostly in the older teenage age group). *"It was a rollercoaster journey, always highly inspiring but sometimes very difficult and challenging."*

"I remember one of my mentees wanted to be taught how to tell the time so that he could keep his appointments. He was too embarrassed to ask for help; afraid that he might be judged for not knowing such a simple thing. An insight into how things which one might take completely for granted might be the cause of so much struggle for another person, just puts everything into perspective."

"We can transfer the learnings from such experiences to primary care, especially in times when there might be a tendency to get frustrated (due to various reasons like language barriers, cultural differences, shortage of time due to appointment time limits), in acknowledging how certain patients might have suffered through unimaginable hardships, and do deserve extra time and compassion."

Dr Elliott also volunteered during the Commonwealth Games in 2022 as a GP in the athletes' village. She recalls numerous fascinating experiences; some of the most memorable ones were providing medical assessments, advice and management for long-term ulcers and infections to athletes arriving from remote islands with no or very limited medical access. She also managed patients with illness contracted after migration for the Games. She was also involved in medical fitness testing for athletes. This involved managing several musculoskeletal concerns and queries regarding permissible medications before competing.

"Meeting, interacting, working with, and hearing the enthralling stories of international athletes and volunteers from various backgrounds was an unforgettable experience, and given the opportunity and the time, I would gladly do it again."

Dr Elliott's advice for volunteer and charity roles:

- **Proactiveness**: contact your local council for awareness regarding different volunteering roles and their requirements, and see what suits you. An online search would be another way to find out and research about volunteering and charity roles.

Continuing professional development and additional qualifications

Dr Elliott is quite the learner, as she doesn't forget to underline the importance of her roles as an educationalist in helping her to sustain her skill set as a trainer and keep it polished and up to date. She finds extra studying very interesting and so makes the time for it: *"I love to keep on my toes, looking stuff up to answer questions, diving deep (!) into my interests and brushing up on the recent advances"*. She also expresses immense gratitude towards the supportive work environment she had over the years. For example, her educational supervisor and programme director helped her prepare for different exams, her colleagues such as the diabetes nurses helped her prepare for the diploma in diabetes care. This helped her to pursue her professional goals and aspirations.

Research, coaching and appraisal roles

Dr Elliott has also been involved with research activities as she was based at a research practice. She completed a research course, following which she became a clinical investigator in the practice. She mentions that she started with research, thinking it would be helpful for the practice, but she realised that she didn't enjoy it, which led her to discontinue the research roles.

Dr Elliott mentioned undertaking coaching courses (she has received coaching as well as having provided coaching sessions) to enhance her other roles.

Dr Elliott was a GP appraiser from 2008 to 2015. She feels it was rewarding to congratulate GPs on their achievements, and it helped her utilise her coaching skill set to encourage and motivate them to work out and realise their career aspirations. Appraising was a grounding experience for her: *"the majority of practices have similar problems, and the more we share, the more we can come up with shared solutions. One goes back to work rejuvenated and with a renewed positivity."*

Dr Elliott's advice for GP appraisers:

- **Support**: training for the role is provided and the role is well-supported
- **Flexible**: an appraiser can opt to do more or less appraisal work as per their preference

- **Seasonal**: although spaced out throughout the year, appraisal work occurs more frequently during the months of January to March
- **Experience**: the role warrants some experience with good consultation and listening skills to be able to work out any hidden agendas.

The pros and cons of a portfolio career

Pros:

- **Flexibility and choices**: the flexibility a portfolio career offers is a definite positive factor. Being your own boss affords you the luxury to make choices to pursue your interests, work around your family's needs, maintain a healthy work–life balance and make alterations and changes along the way.
- **Never say no**: a portfolio career allows you to dip in and out of different roles as per your compatibility with the role and the need of the hour. You can dip your toes in and test the waters before diving in. You can always put a pin into a role for now and investigate it again later.

Cons:

- **Uncertainty and seasonality**: different roles in a portfolio career may be uncertain and seasonal and so the workload as well as income may fluctuate highly during different time periods, which might be stressful (especially if you need to have a fixed income each month, e.g. to pay a loan / mortgage).
- **Paperwork**: portfolio careers may involve a lot of paperwork and require good organisation and prioritisation skills (as well as a good accountant).

Final pieces of advice

- **Back to basics**: full knowledge and confidence in the basics of general practice forms the foundation of any further roles. *"I can't emphasise enough the significance of real grounding and confidence in one's own basic GP skills (including honing of good clinical diagnosis and management skills, good communication and consultation skills) before one can consider taking up any other roles."*
- **Start at grassroots level**: being in a regular role in a supportive practice is more conducive towards helping with additional

qualifications and roles (as study leave and funding are some of the advantages in a regular role, as opposed to a locum role). *"Start within a supportive practice where you can cultivate your special interests, which will let you build on those, and once more established, you can consider developing further and branching out."*

- **Take the first step**: be proactive in asking, researching and finding out about opportunities in areas of your interest.

- **Organisation, prioritisation and setting boundaries**: good organisation and prioritisation skills are essential for a portfolio career, to keep track of what you are doing. Avoid spreading yourself too thinly and set healthy boundaries.

- **Go with the flow**: for a portfolio career one needs to be comfortable with uncertainty. Dr Elliott has found it easier to first follow the regular or full-time GP career path (partner and salaried roles), and then decide to switch to part-time roles or less regular (locum role and other seasonal roles), step-by-step and steadily, to get accustomed to and comfortable with the fluctuating nature of the work and income with a portfolio career.

The future

Some of the roles Dr Elliott hopes to pursue in future include becoming a member of the ARCP (Annual Review of Competence Progression) panel and helping with exam question writing.

Dr Elliott is very happy with her career and advises those considering a portfolio career that it is *"very doable"* and to *"go for it!"*.

6.14 Dr Tara George
Out-of-hours, board member, RCGP advisor and podcaster

Interviewed by Dr Gireesha Verma

Tara George, MBCHB, FRCGP, DCH, DRCOG, DFSRH, PGCert Med Ed

- Salaried GP
- GP trainer and OOH trainer/supervisor
- Medical education and teaching
- External advisor to the RCGP
- Mentor for new GPs

General practice

Dr George decided to pursue her career in general practice after working in a GP rotation as a trainee. After completing her GP training, she started working as a salaried GP for a year, followed by working as a partner in the same practice. Over the years, as she took up further roles, she needed to reduce her GP sessions because these were, sadly, not compatible with her partnership role. She therefore resigned from the practice and worked as a locum GP for a year to be able to efficiently balance all the varied roles. The following year, she joined another practice with the *"aim to convert it to a training practice"*. Here she continues to work four clinical sessions a week, including sessions for contraceptive coils and implants. Thanks to the continued efforts by all the practice team, they are now a well-established training practice.

Out-of-hours

Dr George does an OOH session every alternate week. She is also an OOH trainer/supervisor, which *"gives opportunities for teaching and direct clinical supervision along the way"*. She finds the OOH shifts *"fun and involved"*, helping to practise and keep up to date with medicine in acute and subacute presentations. She is fond of the multidisciplinary team, working with GPs, associate clinical practitioners, nurse practitioners, paramedics and non-clinical staff.

Discussing the advantages of OOH, she mentions that the work pattern enables *"flexibility and better work–life balance"* (providing the ability to choose one's working hours). It also involves *"less administrative work"* (compared to routine general practice). *"The working hours have discrete boundaries, facilitating leaving on time after a shift".*

Thinking about the downside of OOH, Dr George mentions the loss of continuity of patient care.

Mental health CCG board member

Dr George worked as a mental health CCG board member for the GP commissioning of perinatal mental health. She mentions that the challenge was to *"translate clinically important and relevant information into lay language so that non-clinical members could fully understand".* It involved managing government resources to figure out effective solutions. It is essential to be mindful in such roles that *"as a representative of primary care, one is bringing forward the combined opinion of one's peers, and not just one's personal opinion".*

Later on in her practice, she worked in an NHS England role as a perinatal mental health GP champion, delivering education to primary care staff on the topic of perinatal mental health.

External advisor for the RCGP

Dr George contributed to the RCGP peer panel as an external advisor for quality control of ARCP (annual review of competence progression) decisions. *"Having a meticulous eye for detail plus being able to see the holistic big picture are valuable assets for this role".* It is a *"transparent process of presenting an unbiased view effectively, compassionately and with appropriate communication".* This role involves being an external representative for ARCP appeals nationally.

The role is very flexible and encourages utilising learning from other practices.

Teaching

Dr George is passionate about medical education. Her numerous educational roles include (past and present):

- Academic training fellow and phase one tutor, University of Sheffield
- Associate postgraduate (PG) dean, East Midlands Deanery
- Honorary senior lecturer, QMUL
- GP trainer and GP training programme director.

She credits the PG Certificate in Medical Education as being incredibly helpful for these roles. She finds these roles *"fulfilling and helping with CPD, as teaching is learning and keeps one up to date"*.

Medical mentoring

After appropriate training and supervision, Dr George worked as a mentor in the Derbyshire new to practice fellowship scheme for GPs in their initial two years post-CCT to help with transitioning into independent practice.

She has mentored GPs and reminisces about *"mentoring GPs when they felt stuck and needed someone to help them in decision-making to move further in their career"*. She emphasises that the skills in mentoring involve being patient and remembering *"it is about someone else, not about you"*. It is vital to help the mentees make the right decision for them, and not to be influenced by the mentor's personal thoughts and beliefs.

Mentor for the Social Mobility Foundation

Dr George has been mentoring for the SMF, a charity supporting young people from disadvantaged backgrounds. It involves chaperone-supervised Zoom meetings for mentorship, with professionals in the young person's profession of interest, providing motivation and role models. She describes the role as *"valuable and fulfilling, which is flexible and not very time-consuming"*, and encourages others to become involved.

Writing articles and delivering courses

Dr George has been writing educational articles and delivering medical education courses for Don't Forget the Bubbles (a paediatrics medical education resource: dontforgetthebubbles. com). She is the deputy editor for *InnovAiT*. Her advice is to *"stop procrastinating and keep writing to get better at it"*. She believes that writing helps to *"improve communication skills and keeps one up to date"*.

She is an education facilitator and teaches on a Teach the Teacher course for Seventeen Seconds (www.seventeenseconds.co.uk), which is a medical education start-up.

She is a facilitator for Scaling the Heights (scalingtheheights.com) and the director of GP5T, which enables her to organise Continued Professional Development for GP trainers.

The Bedside Reading podcast

Dr George first realised her interest in hosting podcasts after she was interviewed. Dr George believes that *"people are willing to share their experiences, and finding other people doing what one wants to do is always a step in the right direction"*. She is the host of the Bedside Reading podcast, which discusses *"themes from fiction, memoir and other non-traditional non-textbooks which help to make us better at what we do"*.

Pros and cons of a portfolio career

Dr George says the pros of a portfolio career involve *"different opportunities and variety of work which keeps one fresh, never being bored and meeting lots of different people"*.

The cons include *"switching on and off quite rapidly between different roles"* and *"management of the urgency of tasks in various roles"*.

Dr George's final advice for pursuing a portfolio career

- **Prioritisation**: a portfolio career is based on *"effective management and organisation skills"*. *"Recognising what you need to do and what you can outsource helps by allowing you to focus more on the things that matter to you"*. It is also worthwhile *"keeping protected time for certain things"*.
- **Interest**: finding work which brings you *"joy and intellectual satisfaction"* is really fulfilling.
- **Spontaneity**: Dr George says it works better for her to *"go with the flow rather than try to plan everything, as often when desperately goal seeking, one might have really unrealistic ideas of where one is going"*.
- **Taking the leap**: Dr George believes it is important *"not to take oneself too seriously"*, and that *"if you've got an idea, go for it!"*
- **Balancing act**: it's easy to get completely occupied by work. Make sure you have time for yourself and your hobbies. This is essential in finding a healthy *"work–life balance"*.
- **Looping**: *"Once you do a few things, you get asked for other things"*, and it helps with networking and building contacts.

Chapter summary – key pointers from portfolio GPs

You should now have a greater insight into the careers of those living the 'portfolio life'. I hope you have seen what is possible. Importantly, I hope you have realised that each career is unique, like individuals. It takes a significant amount of time to refine one's career, getting the 'right' balance, and this is usually subject to change.

- You can't create a portfolio career without first knowing your 'why'. Why do you want to create a portfolio career?
- Continue to reflect regularly on your interests. The goal is to stay truly passionate about what you are doing. Life is short, so follow your passions.
- If the centre of your portfolio career is general practice, then focus on that first and build a solid foundation.
- There are no shortcuts. You must increase your skill set to build confidence and open up other opportunities for growth.
- It takes time to develop a career you are truly satisfied with. Be patient and keep going.
- A portfolio career that works well is like a jigsaw puzzle with all pieces fitting together seamlessly. Ensure you have a clear direction and some continuity in your career.
- Getting to the next level requires the building of relationships. Network, network, network!
- Opportunities won't necessarily come and find you. Look for and seize opportunities whenever you can.
- Don't always stick to 'the plan'; being spontaneous can take you down interesting avenues.
- Flexibility is important for a portfolio career. How can you create this in your own career? Think about what you would like your working week to look like.
- A portfolio career can be isolating and demanding, and requires some level of risk-taking. You won't get far without prioritising wellbeing and self-care.
- You will need to be organised, committed, innovative, proactive, able to plan carefully – get used to uncertainty and most of all believe in you!
- The recipe to creating your portfolio career lies in truly understanding who you are, establishing your interests and passions coupled with upskilling, networking and the right skills and qualities.

Appendix 1:
Further reading

Almagor, E. (2012) Ctesias and the importance of his writings revisited. *Electrum*, **19:** 9–40.

Baptiste, P. (2015) Mental health issues among medical students. *BMJ Opinion*. Available at: https://blogs.bmj.com/bmj/2015/09/22/patrice-baptiste-mental-health-issues-among-medical-students (accessed 27 August 2024)

Bjerke, M.B. and Renger, R. (2017) Being smart about writing SMART objectives. *Eval Program Plann*, **61:** 125–7.

Bourne, A., Lyons, C. and McCrudden, C. (2016) *Building a Portfolio Career*, 3rd edition. Management Books.

Buranova, D. (2015) The value of Avicenna's heritage in development of modern integrative medicine in Uzbekistan. *Integrative Medicine Research*, **4(4):** 220–4.

Cavanaugh, R. (2017) Dr Girolamo Fracastoro (1478–1553) and the poetry of syphilis. *Journal of Medical Biography*, **25(1):** 60–1.

Clear, J. (2018) *Atomic Habits: tiny changes, remarkable results: an easy and proven way to build good habits and break bad ones*. Penguin Random House.

Cooper, W.H., Graham, W.J. and Dyke, L.S. (1993) Tournament players. *Research in Personnel and Human Resources Management*, **11:** 83–132.

Costa, P.T. and McCrae, R.R. (1992) *Revised NEO Personality Inventory and NEO Five-factor Inventory Professional Manual*. Psychological Assessment Resources.

Davis, J., Wolff, H.-G., Forret, M. and Sullivan, S. (2020) Networking via LinkedIn: an examination of usage and career benefits. *Journal of Vocational Behavior*, **118:** 103396.

de Janasz, S.C. and Forret, M.L. (2008) Learning the art of networking: a critical skill for enhancing social capital and career success. *Organizational Behavior Teaching Review*, **32(5):** 629–50.

Department for Education and The Rt Hon Chris Skidmore (2019) *Graduates continue to benefit with higher earnings*. Available at:

www.gov.uk/government/news/graduates-continue-to-benefit-with-higher-earnings (accessed 27 August 2024)

Department of Health and Social Care (2020) *Mend the Gap: the independent review into gender pay gaps in medicine in England.*

Durlauf, S.N. and Fafchamps, M. (2005) 'Social capital'. Chapter 26 in Aghion, P. and Durlauf, S.N. (eds) *Handbook of Economic Growth*, volume 1, part B, pp. 1639–99. Elsevier.

Echeverría, V.I. (2010) Girolamo Fracastoro and the invention of syphilis. *História, Ciências, Saúde—Manguinhos*, **17(4):** 877–84.

Fischer, L.-P. and Nathalie, S.-T. (2003) Luke, evangelist and physician. *Histoire des Sciences Médicales*, **37.2:** 215–24.

Forth, J., Bryson, A. and Theodoropoulos, N. (2022) Ethnic minority workers earn much less than white counterparts within the same firm. *The Conversation.*

Ginzberg, E., Ginsburg, S.W., Axelrad, S. and Herma, J.L. (1951) *Occupational Choice: an approach to a general theory.* Columbia University Press.

GMC (2013) *Doctors' use of social media.*

Golden, J. (2015) Saint Luke: chronicler of the first Christmas and most published of any doctor. *British Journal of General Practice*, **65(641):** 653.

Gorbatov, S., Khapova, S.N. and Lysova, E.I. (2019) Get noticed to get ahead: the impact of personal branding on career success. *Frontiers in Psychology*, **10:** Article 2662.

Granovetter, M.S. (1973) The strength of weak ties. *American Journal of Sociology*, **78(6):** 1360–80.

Handy C. (1991) *The Age of Unreason*, 2nd ed. Random House Business.

Handy, C. (1995) *The Empty Raincoat: making sense of the future.* Cornerstone.

Higher Education Statistics Agency (HESA) (2022) *Graduate Outcomes 2019/20: summary statistics.* Available at: www.hesa.ac.uk/news/16-06-2022/sb263-higher-education-graduate-outcomes-statistics (accessed 27 August 2024)

HM Government & Saxton Bampfylde. *Reach Mentoring Programme: a guide for mentors and mentees.* Available at: www.saxbam.com/

wp-content/uploads/2019/09/Reach-4.pdf (accessed 27 August 2024)

Holland, J.L. (1997) *Making Vocational Choices*, 3rd ed. Psychological Assessment Resources.

Hopson, B. and Ledger, K. (2019) *And What Do You Do? 10 steps to creating a portfolio career*. A&C Black Publishers.

Iyengar, S., Ehrlich, J., Chung, E. *et al.* (2022) Evaluation of a virtual networking event for emerging women leaders in global health. *Ann Glob Health*, **88(1):** 54.

Kirk, L.M. (2007) Professionalism in medicine: definitions and considerations for teaching. *Proc (Bayl Univ Med Cent)*, **20(1):** 13–16.

Kitchen, E. (2017) What is the value of networking? An examination of trade show attendee outcomes. *Journal of Convention & Event Tourism*, **18(3):** 191–204.

Matthews, R.J. (2017) A theory for everything? Is a knowledge of career development theory necessary to understand career decision making? *European Scientific Journal*, **13(7):** 320–34.

McMahon, M. and Patton, W. (2018) Systemic thinking in career development theory: contributions of the Systems Theory Framework. *British Journal of Guidance & Counselling*, **46(2):** 229–40.

Merrick, L. and Stokes, P. (2008) *Talent Management*. Available at: www.coachmentoring.co.uk/blog/2018/09/talent-management-mentoring (accessed 27 August 2024)

Miller, M. (2020) *My Social Media for Seniors*, 3rd edition. Pearson Education, Inc.

Ng, T.W.H., Eby, L.T., Sorensen, K.L. and Feldman, D.C. (2005) Predictors of objective and subjective career success: a meta-analysis. *Personnel Psychology*, **58(2):** 367–408.

Nimmons, D., Giny, S. and Rosenthal, J. (2019) Medical student mentoring programs: current insights. *Adv Med Educ Pract*, **10:** 113–23.

Office for National Statistics (2023) *Ethnicity Pay Gaps UK*.

Parsons, F. (1909) *Choosing a Vocation*. Houghton Mifflin.

Passmore, J., Peterson, D.B. and Freire, T. (eds) (2013) *The Wiley Blackwell Handbook of the Psychology of Coaching and Mentoring*. John Wiley & Sons Ltd.

Patton, W. and McMahon, M. (2015) The Systems Theory Framework of career development: 20 years of contribution to theory and practice. *Australian Journal of Career Development*, **24:** 141–7.

Preston, S. (2017) *Portfolio Careers: how to work for passion, pleasure & profit!* Steve Preston The Career Catalyst.

Reardon, R.C. (2017) Enhancing self-help career planning using theory-based tools. *Journal of Career Assessment*, **25(4):** 650–69.

Review Body on Doctors' and Dentists' Remuneration (2022) *Fiftieth Report 2022.* Crown copyright.

Risse, L., Farrell, L. and Fry, T.R.L. (2018) Personality and pay: do gender gaps in confidence explain gender gaps in wages? *Oxford Economic Papers*, **70(4):** 919–49.

Sampson, J.P., Jr., Peterson, G.W. and Reardon, R.C. (1989) Counselor intervention strategies for computer assisted career guidance: an information processing approach. *Journal of Career Development*, **16:** 139–54.

Sampson, J.P., Jr., Peterson, G.W., Lenz, J.L. and Reardon, R.C. (1992) A cognitive approach to career services: translating concepts into practice. *Career Development Quarterly*, **41:** 67–74.

Sampson, J.P., Jr., McClain, M.-C., Musch, E. and Reardon, R.C. (2013) Variables affecting readiness to benefit from career interventions. *Career Development Quarterly*, **61:** 98–109.

Seibert, S.E. and Kraimer, M.L. (2001) The five-factor model of personality and career success. *Journal of Vocational Behavior*, **58:** 1–21.

Seibert, S.E., Crant, J.M. and Kraimer, M.L. (1999) Proactive personality and career success. *Journal of Applied Psychology*, **84:** 416–27.

Seibert, S.E., Kraimer, M.L. and Liden, R.C. (2001) A social capital theory of career success. *Academy of Management Journal*, **44:** 219–37.

Stanley, N. (online) *What to do when you want to do everything: is a portfolio career right for you?* Career Shifters. Available at: www.careershifters.org/expert-advice/what-to-do-when-you-want-to-do-everything-is-a-portfolio-career-right-for-you (accessed 27 August 2024)

Sterling, A.D., Thompson, M.E., Wang, S. *et al.* (2020) The confidence gap predicts the gender pay gap among STEM graduates. *Proc Natl Acad Sci USA*, **117(48):** 30303–8.

Stevens, K. and Whelan, S. (2019) Negotiating the gender wage gap. *Industrial Relations*, **58:** 141–88.

Super, D.E. (1953) A theory of vocational development. *American Psychologist*, **8:** 185–190.

Super, D.E. (1990) 'A life-span life-space approach to career development'. In D. Brown and L. Brooks (eds) *Career Choice and Development: applying contemporary theories to practice,* 2nd ed, pp. 197–261. Jossey-Bass.

Svenningsson, J., Höst, G., Hultén, M. and Hallström, J. (2021) Students' attitudes toward technology: exploring the relationship among affective, cognitive and behavioral components of the attitude construct. *Internation Journal of Technology and Design Education*, **32**: 1531–51.

Teoli, D., Sanvictores, T. and An, J. (2023) *SWOT Analysis*. StatPearls.

Trabue, M.R. (1933) Occupational ability patterns. *Personnel Journal*, **11:** 344–51.

Troscianko, E. and Bray, R. (2016, updated 2020) *Portfolio Careers: how to optimise and manage them*. Careers Service, University of Oxford. Available at: www.careers.ox.ac.uk/files/portfolio-careers-workbookpdf (accessed 27 August 2024)

Turner, R.J. (1960) Sponsored and contest mobility and the school system. *American Sociological Review*, **25:** 855–67.

van Harreveld, F., Nohlen, H. and Schneider, I. (2015) The ABC of Ambivalence: Affective, Behavioral, and Cognitive consequences of attitudinal conflict. *Advances in Experimental Social Psychology*, **52**: 285.

Wils, T., Wils, L. and Tremblay, M. (2014) Revisiting the career anchor model: a proposition and an empirical investigation of a new model of career value structure. *Relations Industrielles / Industrial Relations*, **69(4):** 813–38.

Xu, D. and Fletcher, J. (2016) 'Understanding the relative value of alternative pathways in postsecondary education: evidence from the state of Virginia'. In Shah, M. and Whiteford, G. (eds) *Bridges, Pathways and Transitions: international innovations in widening participation*. Chandos Publishing.

Appendix 2:
Social media tips

- **Create strong and varied passwords** – when signing up to social media sites it might be very tempting to use the same password across different accounts. However, if one account is at risk then others become so too. By extension, you should think twice about using one social media account to log into another one. Longer passwords with a mixture of letters, numbers and special characters are advised (indeed, most websites and apps insist on this by default). Passwords you use regularly will naturally be remembered, but others will be forgotten unless you keep them written down (somewhere secure of course!). Alternatively you could make use of a password manager such as Bitwarden.

- **Don't share personal information when posting** – this includes your date of birth, your phone number, address (think carefully about including your location when posting too). You might also want to be careful with posting potential answers to the typical security questions you get asked for other accounts. Examples are your mother's maiden name, your primary school, your pet's name. Also think carefully about how much information you provide to the platform when creating your account (there is always the possibility of data breaches!).

- **Think carefully about what you post** – since the internet (and your social media accounts) are not private, consider exactly what you post on your profile and in response to other people's posts when commenting. You might be surprised who is watching what you share, and you might even forget who you are connected to! I always try to contribute positively to both the online and offline world, not simply because I know the internet is public or because nothing is truly deleted, but because I genuinely want to make a positive contribution to the world.

- **Think carefully before sharing the contacts in your phone with the social media sites** – many platforms ask for access to the contacts in your phone to see if any of your contacts are using the same platform. This may lead to advertisements (or worse) being sent to those contacts. Furthermore, consider the need for (and potential harm of) downloading additional applications linked to the app (third parties) and games within the app – these can access any sensitive information you have added to your account.

- **Review your privacy and security settings** – consider setting your profiles to private rather than public. There are various settings you can change if you decide you do not want a public profile. For example, with one setting on LinkedIn you can post publicly, but in order for connections to gain access to your complete profile they have to send you a connection request. This may allow for you to 'vet' or check who you are allowing to access your profile. Of course this is not a failsafe approach, but might be a place to start if you are unsure. You can also review your connections regularly; you may want to remove or block connections as you feel necessary.